Capoeira Over 40

How to Be Successful When Starting Capoeira at a Later Age

Chris Roel

© 2017 by **Chris Roel**

All Rights Reserved. No part of this publication may be reproduced in any form or by any means, including scanning, photocopying, or otherwise without prior written permission of the copyright holder.

First Printing, 2017

Printed in the United States of America

Liability Disclaimer

By reading this document, you assume all risks associated with using the advice given below, with a full understanding that you, solely, are responsible for anything that may occur as a result of putting this information into action in any way, and regardless of your interpretation of the advice.

Make sure you are healthy enough for exercise. We are in no way liable for any injury accrued by any parties by doing the exercises, diets, or behaviors described in this book.

Terms of Use

You are given a non-transferable, "personal use" license to this product. You cannot distribute it or share it with other individuals.

Also, there are no resale rights or private label rights granted when purchasing this document. In other words, it's for your own personal use only.

Capoeira Over 40

How to Be Successful When Starting Capoeira at a Later Age

Table of Contents

Introduction..................................9
1. Focus on Fundamentals...............11
2. Modifications...........................19
3. Playing Upright........................27
4. Supplemental Training...............31
5. Diet.......................................37
6. Rest......................................45
7. Yoga.....................................49
8. Music, Language, Culture............51
9. Balancing Life.........................53
10. Conclusion............................55
Thanks For Reading......................57
About the Author........................58
Appendix..................................59

Introduction

You don't have to be 40 years of age to read this book. I was 26 when I first started training Capoeira, but I felt like I was 40. I was 20 pounds overweight, had a pot belly, a double chin, and dwindling daily energy. I felt I had to do something in my life to make a change. Brazilian Capoeira saved my life and helped me chose better acquaintances which ultimately led me improving my life ten times over.

I initially tried regular exercise like running and weights, but something had happened to my metabolism after the age of 25. To make a long story short, I lost 20 pounds in two months, gained flexibility, amazing core strength, positive upbeat goal-orientated friends, and learned a new culture that would continue to inspire me until today.

This book will talk about safe modifications of exercises, diet changes, seeking training partners, conservative style of play and other topics that will show you that you can enjoy Capoeira at any age and be successful.

If you haven't seen my free video series on Capoeira over 40 you can see that here:

http://bit.ly/cap40

This video series will hit the main points and give some great visual tips and exercises. The pages ahead, however, will really delve into how to be successful when starting Capoeira at a later age. Whether 40, 50, 30, or 26, the point is if you feel too out of shape for Capoeira; think again.

Well, I don't want to spend too much time ranting and hollering, so without further ado, let's get started. See you in the next chapter.

Chapter 1
Focus on the Fundamentals

When most people think of Capoeira, they think of the amazing flips and acrobatics. They believe that they too have to flip and fly in the roda, but this is not true. There are hundreds of Mestres and high level Capoeira practitioners that have a smooth game and don't ever go aerial. They focus on fundamentals like deep base, straight kicks, ground movements, and mandinga (sneakiness and playfulness).

So, when starting Capoeira at a later age, you too, should focus on the fundamentals. Learn all your basic dodges. Some of them can be pretty challenging in their own right. For example the Esquiva (frontal) is essentially a giant lunge with one hand on the floor and the other blocking your head. Capoeiristas pass in and out of this position effortlessly and smoothly.

I admit when I first started training this was one of most demanding moves, although fundamental. Pretty soon my legs started getting stronger, and I was able to pass in and out of this position fairly easily.

Developing a great base or cadeira position is also key. This will help you resist takedowns, and make yours more solid. You will still be developing your base long after you begin training. It gets stronger each year if you maintain you training and playing in rodas.

Kicks
Next, focus on straightening your kicks. Capoeira has a very nice aesthetic to it because of its associated circular kicks. They are like no other martial arts' kicks because they aren't chambered. They are stiff with locked leg, and moved by the torso. They do have other kicks that are chambered, but the three main kicks, Quexada, Armada, and Meia Lua de Compasso, are not.

Take the time to straighten them. Here's on exercise you can do. Stand next to the wall or stretching bar. With your outside foot locked with toes flexed back towards you, perform circles with your leg, first going forward then finishing behind you. Your leg should be straight as can be. Do as many as you can (at least 20), and then switch legs. When switching legs, you should turn around and face the other way so that leg performing he exercise is the one furthest away from the wall.

Acrobatics
Now let's back up a bit. Don't think you will be flying across the room. Even kids who start training Capoeira start at the fundamental level. I have had several students struggle with getting their bridge, or even their bridge push-up. No worries. As long as you can Ginga, kick, and dodge you will be okay.

This is Capoeira, so of course never stop trying to get your bridge. Back flexibility will help you most in Capoeira when trying to perform either aerial or ground acrobatics. The bridge is the first thing you need to master before trying to move on. Lay on your back bend your knees with flat feet close to your bottom. Put your hands by your ears flat palms on the floor, with elbows up and fingers facing you. Then push up to the bridge. Doesn't work? Then try using your head as support to gain a little height, then try to push up again. The goal is to be able to do 20 solid bridge push-ups with navel high in the air. Start with 10, then move to 15, and then 20. You also will want to perform 20 second bridge holds. Push up into bridge and hold it as high as you can for 20 seconds. Do at least three reps.

Don't get discouraged if you can't do it. Get a partner to help you. Slowly ween yourself off a spotter as you get stronger. It could take you a long time, but don't give up. If you are really trying and busting your rump, then you should make real progress in no time.

The Aú, or Capoeira cartwheel, is another acrobatic fundamental. Just start low, and slowly raise your level as your upper body gets stronger. This is a direct reflection of your handstand strength, so make sure you are dedicating time to your handstands on the wall or with a spotter. Capoeira is amazing in that it strengthens your body in so many ways. Once again, don't get discouraged if you're not making fast progress in your acrobatics. You'll need to build your upper body strength. It could take more time if you are weaker in your upper body. You don't have to lift weights, but maybe some pushups and other body weight exercises can help, like dips.

The Queda de Rins, or elbow balance, is another tough ground maneuver. Push it out. In <u>O Rei's Capoeira Ground Game System</u>, I mention that 80 year old yoga grandmas can do this move, so you can too. Check out the modification chapter to see how to fake it until you make it. Pretty much you're going to have to just grit through it. I tell my students that there is just you and the floor. There's no secret except you and hard work. Once you get this one, you'll have a great feeling of accomplishment.

Movement

With these fundamentals and some basic movement combinations, you will pretty much be a functional Capoeira player. Don't sell your self short. Remember, there are younger people who fail by not trying. Don't let that be you. You are wiser, more experienced in life and know the value of perseverance. Try the following exercises and just perfect these. Anyone, regardless of age can perform these, just stay with it.

- Rolé to both sides from Base (cadeira)
- Esquiva to Rolé both sides
- Esquiva to Negativa to Rolé both sides'
- Esquiva to Negativa to Escapa
- Circular Kicks land to the Base Rolé

For any of these basic maneuvers, you can substitute Aú instead of Rolé if you're feeling up to it, but you don't have to. You can navigate your game as a beginner with these moves alone and still look competent.

Well, we've covered a lot in just the beginning chapter, so go back over it if you need to. Remember, there's a lot of these goodies in the FREE Video series "Capoeira Over 40", so make sure to check that out. See you in the next chapter.

Chapter 2
Modifications

So we learned in chapter 1 that we must concentrate on the fundamentals, no matter what age we are. In this chapter, I'm going to give you some tips to modify some exercises if you happen to be having trouble with them. Now we all had trouble with them. There will have to be a waiting period for your body to get stronger before you start accomplishing moves 100%. If you start feeling that you are taking to long to get them then here are some tips. That judgement is up to you.

I've had students take years to get their bridge. I took 3 months to get into it and another month to get out of it. Work hard but make sure you are having fun. Capoeira is very rewarding on so many levels. Don't let some measly obstacle prevent you from having fun with Capoeira. Persevere, work hard, and accomplish!

Let's first talk about the Queda De Rins (QDR)--that elbow balance that 80 year Yoga grandmas do. It is harder than it looks, but it's mostly about structural balance instead of strength. Yes, at first you will use a lot of strength until you find that sweet spot of balance, but when you do get it, you'll know what I'm talking about. That being said, you will also have to condition you wrist for the extra pressure in this move. Don't wimp out. It will go away in time, unless you have a wrist injury. These ground acrobatics will really strengthen your wrists and ligaments, so stick with it!

Ideally, in the basic QDR balled up position, you have your near hand flat palm on the floor with elbow at 90 degrees straight up into either your hip or rib cage. The side of your head can be on the floor and your far hand is extended in front of your face palm down on the floor. Your knees are tucked into your chest with hips forward, not down. You are completely balanced in the air on your tripod of appendages--head and two palms.

This is the way to modify the position until you gain enough balance, wrist flexibility, and strength to perform it fully. Everything is the same, except that you can leave you feet slightly touching the floor. This will relieve some of the pressure and weight from the rest of your supports. Make sure to really strike the QDR pose, engaging your wrists, and placing that elbow in the hip or ribs. This will get you by until you really get the balance/strength.

Next, we're going to talk about the handstand, or bananeira. Mostly this is strength but when trying to walk on hands, you'll need more balance. In my school we usually spot a beginner doing a handstand next to the wall with their back against the wall when upside down. The spotter will elongate the spine and arms by pulling up on the legs of the student. Once a student has built up enough strength to do it him/herself, he/she will kick up to the wall with no spotter.

Here's how to modify this exercise if you're having trouble kicking up into your handstand on the wall. Start facing away from the wall and with your hands on the floor, back up until your feet touch the wall.

Then climb up the wall backwards, walking your feet higher and higher until you're all the way chest flat against the wall. Don't worry, if you feel scared or weak, just go as high as you feel comfortable. Do your twenty-second holds if you can. If you can't do that, build your way up to it, starting with 10-second holds.

As a precaution, here is the safe way to exit this modified wall hand stand. Instead of walking back down, which could take a lot more strength and energy, kick your feet to the side as if finishing a cartwheel (Aú). This will bring you off the wall safely when you're fatigued.

Next, is the Ponte, or bridge. Ideally, a student should be able to push up into the bridge after a few weeks, and rotate into it in about 3-6 months, however, this book is called "Capoeira Over 40" for a reason. This will challenge many students, young and old, so don't get discouraged. As mentioned in the last chapter, there are students who take years to get their bridge. It just depends on your beginning upper-body strength, age, and beginning flexibility. I had horrible flexibility when I first started training Capoeira, and it changed my life. Don't give up on your bridge, because once you get your bridge you can move on to some pretty amazing moves. It's all about the back flexibility. Here is the way to modify it if you're having trouble making gains on your Ponte.

Laying on your back in preparation for your Capoeira bridge, you will bring your feet close to your body, knees bent, and arch up pushing your hips off the floor. This should create enough room for you to get your palms in proper bridge position. Use your traps to pivot on and then your head, as you climb up higher. Now it's time to engage your arms. Once your hands are in bridge position, perform your bridge push up, even if it's just one inch off the floor.

Do ten 1-inch bridge pushups, or as many as you can. Each time you do your bridge pushups, try to go higher and higher with each session. The ultimate goal is to push up all the way with arms fully extended twenty times, or a twenty-second hold. I won't even talk about the bridge rotation, because once you can do 20 bridge push ups you'll be ready for <u>O Rei's Capoeira Ground Game System</u>.

Next, is the Aú, or Capoeira cartwheel. We'll talk further about the Aú in chapter 4, however here is away to modify the Capoeira cartwheel when first learning. Some people don't have enough upper body strength. Some people don't have enough core strength for getting their legs over their head. Some people don't have enough coordination and trip themselves up when performing. Or...some people have all these problems or a combination of them.

Here is a way to modify the Aú if you are having problems. First, you must know how to do a Rolé. Do the Rolé, but add a small jump instead. Do this exercise back and forth to get the correct leg coordination. Pretty soon you'll be jumping high, and then ultimately doing Aú.

Next, we're going to talk about Macaco, the monkey flip. Most people do the following anyway, and it's totally okay. Starting in cocorinha (macaco position), initiate the macaco but do an Aú instead. This happens when you turn your hips to the front instead of going over the top. The ultimate goal of the Macaco is to go over the top, but don't sweat the details on this one. Students take years to go over the top, and others get it in a couple months.

To wrap up the chapter, just train safely and modify any movements where pain is experienced. Ask your instructor for more tips. See you in the next chapter.

Chapter 3
Playing Upright is Still Cool

When most people think of Capoeira, they think of amazing acrobatics, flips, and turning inside out on the floor. You don't have to do this to have a nice game in the roda. If you are starting at a later age, I'm going to give you a couple tips to play smoothly while staying upright.

These are the recommended fundamentals you should at least have a good understanding of:

- Circular Kicks: (Quexada, Armada, MLC)
- Straight Kicks (Bencão, Martelo, Pisão)
- Rolé (Aú or Macaco optional)
- Escapa or Giro de Costa
- All dodges (Quebrada all Esquivas)
- A good Base or Cadeira

That's not too much to ask. When you can blend these together nicely and have a good conversation, that's all you need. There are hundred's of masters who just use these alone. Once a Capoeira player grows old, he too wants to enjoy the beautiful game of the roda. I'll give you some mini-sequences you can dress up with style and use to make your simple game beautiful.

Sequence 1:
Esquiva Left, Quebrada, Esquiva Left, and then back to Base and Ginga.

Dress this up with some bounce and hand gestures to make it smoother. Go deeper in you base as you get familiar with it. This can be used anytime some kicks at you, or just as a way to buy time.

Sequence 2:
Esquiva Lateral Left, Esquiva Lateral Right, and finally Esquiva Lateral Left before returning back to Ginga.

Once again, add some bounce to this movement. It will appear you are swaying back and forth, but it's actually a functional dodge and a tricky set up.

Sequence 3:
Fake Meia Lua de Compasso, Escapa, Look left, Look right, Exit any side.

This is very good sneaky and stylish. The three sequences are a great simple addition to your game. I usually teach these sequences during our Benguela month. Benguela is a type of Capoeira game that's more funky, stylistic, and closer than Regional or Contemporenea.

Then you can always play fight style if the music dictates it, but that's outside the scope of this book. You should learn from a qualified instructor your Capoeira martial arts. This is no substitute to a Capoeira group, only supplemental training. If you live too far away from a Capoeira group, you may want to check out some of my other training systems at www.gingaandgrowstrong.com

The point is that you don't have to do back flips or turn inside out to have a nice game in the roda. It doesn't matter if you are older, you can still have fun in Brazilian

Capoeira, by playing upright. See you in the next chapter.

Chapter 4
Supplemental training/Partner Work

The reason I came up with "Capoeira over 40" was that one of my followers from India sent me an email regarding one of my digital training systems. He said he loved the system, however, he was concerned that because he was 40 years old and overweight, he was unsure how far he could advance in my ground game system.

I assured him that he would do great, and that I too started training Capoeira 20 pounds over weight. I also told him that I would produce a free video series and send it to him. That's where the the video series with tips to be successful in Capoeira came rom. If you haven't seen the series, click here

http://bit.ly/cap40

In the third video I explain that training with a partner is very beneficial. Many people who buy my products do not have access to a traditional Capoeira academy, so to keep growing, I recommend that they seek out a training partner. Even if you are a member of an official

Capoeira group, it is good too training with a partner outside the academy.

If you feel that you may be too old or out of shape for Capoeira, I have several students over 40 training with me at my academy in Corpus Christi and even a 50+ student. Training with a partner outside the studio is what you need to nail down the techniques you're having trouble with in class. You need to train by yourself also, but the synching up, takedowns, and playful aspects can only be learned by practicing with a partner.

In a later chapter we're going to talk about sufficient rest, but you want to plan into your training regimen some outside solo and partner training. I am going to give you some basic partner training exercises that are extremely beneficial. This book's aimed at the older beginner Capoeira practitioner, however, I will touch on some older intermediate issues later in the book. Let's move on to the partner exercises.

Weaving Quexadas, Armadas and Meia Lua de Compasso

As mentioned into first video, a beginner should concentrate on basic fundamentals. For example, the first partner exercise we're going to work on is weaving Quexadas. Gaining flexibility and good form in your legs is important, and achievable by anyone, of any age or shape.

The exercise is as follows:

•Partner One turns sideways in quebrada position and initiates the Quexada. (For a full description of check out my Fundamentals of Brazilian Capoeira OR access the bonus area for free) Bonus area:

•Partner Two dodges with quebrada and initiates a Quexada crossing partner One. This continues for at least 20 repetitions. Then increase speed and proximity as you gain experience.

Keep your legs locked and toes flexed back. Once you start, there is no more ginga-ing. When performing the same exercise with Armada and Meia Lua de Compasso, you will perform the sequence going left, then right, then left…etc. There will be a half a ginga in between each kick. This will give control of your kicks and confidence in exchanging in the roda. You can move on to Armada and MLC one you are ready.

Dodging with a Partner Kicking

Next, Esquiva Negativa Rolé with a partner. If you have knee problems, go slowly, but this is a good one to strengthen your leg muscles, and ultimately read your opponents body language to escape in style. We'll start easy with just a a simple kick, Passa Pé (Meia Lua de Frente).

- Match up your ginga with your partner
- Partner One will perform a Passa Pé
- Partner Two will dodge with esquiva, transition to negativa, then escape with Rolé

You can use this exercise with any kick: Quexada, Armada, Meia Lua de Compasso, Ponta Pé (martelo) or just do it in the roda for style and movement

Push Kick Drill with a Partner

Finally, a simple Benção drill that allows you to train safely, yet still learn how to kick your opponent.

Standing in a long room or outdoors, face your partner. You will lift you leg and place your foot on the chest of you partner. Then explode by pushing your partner back with the bottom of your foot. When done correctly, it should not hurt your partner. Don't snap the kick. Merely, make contact with your foot securely, then push forcefully. The only way your opponent will get hurt is if he/she falls down and hits themselves.

Partner Two should keep their abs flexed and brace for the kick. Once you have decent control with this kick, you can move on to some of the more advanced kicks: Pisão, Chapa Giratoria, and others.
That's the beauty of Capoeira. It utilizes dodges instead of blocks and push kicks instead of blocks and lets that practitioner have longevity in their sport.

As we wrap up this chapter, one more thing. When courting a training partner, remember to be respectful. They may not be as hard core as you, so save the head kicks and hard takedowns for someone who wants to train hard. Just be upfront and ask them if they want to train a little bit harder. You do't want to scare away you precious training partner in a very beautiful art form. See you in the next chapter.

Access your book bonuses here:
http://bit.ly/Cap40Bonus

Chapter 5
Diet and Supplements

Along with sufficient rest, the diet is extremely important in meeting your Capoeira and health goals. A big question sometimes encountered is the belly getting in the way of some Capoeira exercises. Others can navigate any move despite the bigger midsection. You can see it on the internet, heavily overweight Capoeira players doing amazing feats.

For most other people, you are going to have to diet and live the Capoeira lifestyle. Most diets fail because they are thought of as just a temporary fasting for an event of some sort. After the beach season, wedding, etc., the person puts back on all their weight and sometimes even more.

You have to change your lifestyle. Exercise, eat healthy, cut down on your alcohol intake, and start hanging out with people with similar goals. You may not be trying to lose weight, but a good diet will help your body perform better and recover faster. You'll have a clearer mind and feel better overall.

Popular Diets For Active Lifestyles (Athletes And Martial Artists)

Diet and Fitness are synonymous terms, but not so much when it comes to Active lifestyles and diet. It is imperative that athletes and other martial artists carefully select their diet. Interestingly, different disciplines have dissimilar habits primarily. A martial artist's diet clearly focuses on local foods accessibility which is extremely important as diet impacts their performance.

Let's take a look at some researched facts about the different types of food our past and present martial artists eat.

Shaolin Monks

The Shaolin Monks' diet is derived from the concept of Buddhism such as pacifism and simplicity. Whatever they eat is geared towards providing the body with the needed energy as well as for spiritual motives.

- **Their diet mainly comprises rice, fruits and vegetables**
  The martial artists are vegetarians since one of the basic tenets of Buddhism endorses pacifism.

- **Raw or steamed Food**
  They eat their food mostly raw or steamed, the simpler the better. Fats and artificial sugars are deliberately not added to their meals.
- **Abstain from dairy and meat**

Soy products like seitan and tofu and also soybeans supplies their protein needs. Meat is also substituted with nuts.

Bruce Lee

Our legendary Bruce Lee cared a great deal about his diet. Any foods that could remotely interfere with his training or performance were completely avoided.

- **Protein shakes**
  Bruce took protein shakes a lot as well as supplements like
  royal jelly, ginseng and vitamins.
- **Low protein, heavy carb diet**
  He depended on carbs mostly for energy as opposed to fats and proteins. However, the carbs were got from rice and vegetables just like the Shaolin monks.
- **Small but frquent meals all through the day**

He ate as much as four to five meals daily to have the energy
for his workouts and performances.
- **No coffee**
He preferred tea to coffee. Green tea has been shown to contain active ingredients that improves and speeds up metabolism.

The Gracie Diet
The Gracie family of Jiu-Jitsu fighters from Brazil sure know how to supply the needed fuel for their intense martial arts training.
- **Spaced out meals**
According to Rorion Gracie, 4 1/2 hours interval between meals is ideal. A martial artist is only allowed to take water between meals.
- **One starch per meal**
Just to keep refueling your energy otherwise you get slow and groggy. A martial artist needs just enough carbs for energy.
- **NO to soda or desserts**
Gracie is of the opinion that people consume too much sugar which is unhealthy for the body.
-

Ronda Rousey
Ronda was famous for Judoka and also a MMA

champion. She is very watchful of her post workout meals. She also varies her diet when aiming at shedding some weight.

- **High carb breakfast**

Rousey typically kick starts her day with oatmeal or other sources of high carb. It supplies her with the energy she needs to get going.

- **High carb/half protein lunch and High protein dinner**
  She also supplements her intake of protein with probiotic drinks and protein shakes.
- **Snacks**
  She snacks on almonds, trail mix and frozen grapes.
- **No meals before sleeping.**
  Rousey takes her last meal at least 3 hours before going to sleep.

Fabricio Werdum

Fabricio Werdum (BJJ intensive and renowned MMA fighter) eats more of carbohydrates and protein. He sure puts it to good use with his heavyweight class fights, so the calories don't get to waste!

- **Low carb**
  His carb meal sources include fruits, toast and a little amount of rice only. His energy mostly comes from fat and protein Paleo-esque diet.
- **Lots of protein**

Protein is a constant in his meals. It could be from protein
shakes, grilled chicken or other protein sources.

• **Many meals**

He tries to take 8 meals every day but also supplements with light meals and protein shakes.

Diet is an integral aspect of your physical and mental training. The focus should be on eating just the right amount and combination of nutrients to refuel your energy.

Everyone is different and should consult their physician or dietician ideally, for best results. Everyone should determine which diet works best for them and integrate into their lives. Yes, there will be cheat days, and some tough days, but stick with it. Over time it will become your lifestyle

Supplements

First, make sure your'e taking your daily supplements. Either your one a day from the local pharmacy or they have the multi-vitamin packs at your supplement store. Make sure to do research on each multivitamin. They are usually for active people. You will be running your metabolism, cycling out water, vitamins, and waste more rapidly as you exercise more in your life.

I also recommend fish oils (Omega-3's) for good cardiovascular and joint health. Any other joint and ligament care supplements, I recommend you investigating. It's worth it.

Protein and Recovery

No you don't have to be a body builder to drink protein shakes. They are very official in your rebuilding of muscles you will be rip in Capoeira practice. There are other sups you can take: branch chain amino acids, creatine, and others. My bench press max jumped 40 pounds in high school by taking creatine phosphate. Of course I worked hard, but the recovery supplement made a huge difference.

Water

Make sure you are drinking enough water. Quit the sodas, sweet tea, and other sugary drinks. They are useless to you. Mind over matter, cold turkey those deadly drinks. You can also drink coconut water. It's great for hydrating your body and has a nice taste.

The bottom line is, whatever, diet you choose:

- to eat smaller meals more frequetly
- Watch your carbs
- Stay hydrated
- Quit or Cut down on sodas, sugary drinks, and alcohol
- Eat more fruits and vegetables
- Take daily supplements and possibly protein and recovery drinks

For a more detailed description on healthy dieting and Capoeira healthy lifestyle, look out for my upcoming book "Eat and Ginga Strong"

Chapter 6
Rest

It is recommended by the National Sleep Foundation that adults ages18-25 and ages 26-65 get 7-9 hours of sleep per day. This also depends on you activity level thought out the day, and your week. When I first started training, I took 2 classes a week, and ran , lifted weights 2-3 times a week on my off days. I wasn't' on shape at all, but rather 20 pounds overweight with a potbelly and double-chin. I definitely had some work to do ahead of me.

Within 2 months, I lost 20 pounds and became shredded. I definitely got my rest, going to bed around 9-10 PM each night. I woke up around 5-6 AM every boring depending if my infant son was awake or not.

Rest is extremely important in your Capoeira development and longevity. Don't go out drinking all night and plan on getting up early. Your personal and professional life are on the line too. You don't want to be so tired you'll miss work and get fired, or miss breakfast with you spouse.

(But if you're pushing 40, then you already know that life lesson)

The one thing about martial arts and Capoeira specifically, is that it encourages a healthy lifestyle of exercise, self-discipline, healthy diet, and abstinence from alcohol and drugs. Keep a clean well rested engine, and your body will thank you for it.

If you don't do any other physical activity, I recommend to train 3-5 times a week for a few months until your body gets used to it. Then listen to your body and re-assess how many time you need. If you're active already, then I recommend 2-3 times a week and if you're hungry for more then add another class or two per week.

As you get in better shape, your body will be able to handle more, but don't sacrifice quality for quantity. Don't train 5 times a sweet and show up useless to class. Instead, train 2-3 times a week focused, energetic, and well rested. You'll make more progress that way, especially if you're thin to conquer a new move.

Batizado Week
The way Capoeira groups give ranks are in event called Batizados. They are baptisms, or welcoming in of new students in to the Capoeira community. They're usually composed

of a weekend of workshops by goest instructors, and the celebration and qualification of advancing students. These are extremely fun events where you will meet new visiting students from all over the state, country, and sometimes world.

You will be training several house fro two days, with little rest. You may be housing visitors from out of town and networking with a new positive crowd. These events are fun, yet draining. On the Sunday ending the weekend you may just be laying in bed all day recovering. As you experience more, you will have more energy to get up and have brunch with your new friends as you see them off, or some go futon the town for one last tourist activity before going back home.

Regardless, you'll have to manage your rest and recovery in relation to your fitness level.

- Don't go out Friday night. (Workshops are in the morning)
- Stay hydrated all weekend
- Go out Saturday to mingle with your new friends if you can…if not get some rest

- Sunday sleep it in until you can get up and see your friends off

- Have fun!

Chapter 7
Yoga

Namaste! I first got into Yoga because I started training Brazilian Jiu-Jitsu. It stiffened my odd so much that it almost undid everything that Capoeira had done for me. When training Capoeira by itself, I felt I had no need for Yoga. I bought it was a aster back. Well, I'm glad I got into it, because it couldn't be further from the the truth. It definitely helps and is a great supplemental training for Capoeira. The meditative aspect and the flexibility aspect are the two factors that had me switching my opinion.

Yoga can be used as a pre-warm up, a cool down, or use throw it in your training regiment on off days. I do Yoga Monday through Friday at 5 AM on Youtube and an additional class on Sundays at a local studio. It helps me reclaim some of my lost flexibility and gain flexibility in ways I hadn't had before.

When I started teaching 3 Capoeira classes a day, I lost some flexibility and some moves from not gaining as much as I would like. Yoga helped me reclaim and reset my flexibility form BJJ. After grappling, I am extremely stiff and need the stretch.

It opens up you hips, back , shoulders and any other body part you want to target. Also, many times in Capoeira class, stretching gets neglected. I know it does in my studio. Although I try to do some could down stretching, as much as I can, there's just too much to teach. Stretching usually takes a back seat. I will include a Yoga for Capoeira sequence in your book bonus area. You can access it by going here:

http://bit.ly/Cap40Bonus

As an older beginner, Yoga will help you increase your flexibility an balance outside of class. Give it a go. I know you won't be disappointed.

Chapter 8
Music, Language, and Culture

There is so much to enjoy in Capoeira that it doesn't always have to be physical. As older students, we shouldn't expect to rain as hard as the 20 year olds, unless you know you're in tip top shape. Enjoy the camaraderie. Enjoy the music and language learning. It's a new culture, so take time to immerse yours in it. Read books on Capoeira and Brazilian history. I recommend "The Little Capoeira Book" by Nestor Capoeira, and any of Mestre Accordeon's (Bira Almeida) books. Study Capoeira music online. Buy a Brazilian Portuguese book to learn more Portuguese. Buy your own instruments and practice at home or outside of class,

Capoeira is truly a rich art. Don't limit yourself by thinking it's purely physical. When I got hurt, I would still show up to class and practice music and cheer on my classmates. Many students stop attending class if they get hurt. Capoeira events in other cities. Take a trip to Brazil to train. A note on traveling:

There is an etiquette to traveling when you belong to an official Capoeira group. Make sure you ask your instructor first. He/She will tell you where a good academy to train in is , whatever city you are visiting. This goes for a Brazil trip too. Don't just get up and fly to Brazil to train if you don't; know anybody there. Safety first. It's not about micromanaging you.

You instructor has been around longer and knows more about safe places and friendly groups. Most groups are ver friendly and have open arms to visitors, but there are a few that just want to blast the new visitor.
If you don't belong to a Capoeira group, its always nice to try to contact the instructor of the academy that you are going to visit to make sure it's a good time. Just show respect, and everything will be alright. Don't be so narrow minded when thinking about your Capoeira development, training, and journey. Learn the language, learn the music, learn the culture, and have fun!

The physical part is just on aspect of this amazing art.

Chapter 9
Balancing Life

As an older human being, we have other issues like kids, mortgages, bills, injuries, spouses, aging relatives, and other issues that young younger counterparts don't. You may have more disposable income and want to take a vacation 3 times a year. That's okay. You may need to take your wife to that winery for your anniversary. You may need to take your son to New York when he graduates high school or college. These are al things that happen in our lives that we shouldn't neglect.

Adopting a health lifestyle of exercise, diet, family, recreation, spirituality, and your professional advancement is key. Make sure that everything is balanced and you are setting goals regularly. Think ahead when planing vacations, Capoeira trips, birthdays, training, and other events. Use a calendar. It will become your best friend if you don't use one already.

If you want to live, breath, eat, and sleep Capoeira, go ahead. The key is consistency. Don't take off for two months. Take off a week and come back swinging instead. If you're trying to advance in rank in your group, have a conversation with your instructor about what it takes and how that fits into your life schedule. Every group is different .

"Everything in moderation" is my philosophy.

Chapter 10
Conclusion

Okay, let's recap the "Capoeira Over 40' lifestyle. Safety first, make sure you're healthy enough for exercise. See a physician if your unsure. Focus on fundamentals like kicks, dodges, bridges, light acrobatics, etc. Use the modifications I have provided to get you by until you get strong enough. Adapt your style of play to your abilities. Play upright and use mandinga. You don't have to flip and fly. Use a training partner to help you with your trouble spots. Also, don't scare him/her off my being too rough or vigorous.

Make sure you watch your diet and take your daily supplements. You can use some of the recommendations I provided or seek out your own through your dietitian or physician. Make sure you are getting enough rest daily and weekly.We're older and have to be sensitive to the issue. Consider integrating Yoga into your training regimen for recovery, warm-up, cool down or flexibility enhancement.

Remember, Capoeira is not purely physical. Study the music, language, culture, and travel, meet new fiends and network through Capoeira. It's a beautiful community. I have Capoeira friends all over the world. Some I've never met, yet we share the common bond of Capoeira, dance, Samba, and enjoying the beautiful vibrant Brazilian culture.

Also remember to keep a balanced life, training, family, spiritual, rest, diet, leisure, and professional. If you use this as a guide, you should navigate you Capoeira journey well, despite being older or out of shape. I hope this guide helped. Make sure to check out the bonus section of this book by clicking

http://bit.ly/Cap40Bonus

Stay blessed my beautiful peeps. Axé

Thanks for Reading!

One last thing. Hey guys I hope you enjoyed my work. To show my appreciation, like always, I have included a book bonus area with videos, Yoga sequences for Capoeira, sample diet, and more! I only ask that rate my book on Amazon. I greatly appreciate your feedback- good and bad. Capoeira has changed my life and set me on a personal improvement journey which I'm still on today. I hope it does at least half of that to you. If you have any comments or questions you can direct them at contact@capcorpus.com Thanks again!

Book Bonus Link: http://bit.ly/Cap40Bonus

About the Author

Chris Roel started training Brazilian Capoeira in 2006 in San Antonio Texas under the guidance of Mestrando Advogado. He has owned and operated Capoeira studios all over Texas and currently resides in Corpus Christi, Texas. He has published over 5 books and 4 digital training systems, two of which hit #1 on Amazon. He started training BJJ in 2014 in Gracie Barra BJJ. See more of his products and blog at www.gingaandgrowstrong.com

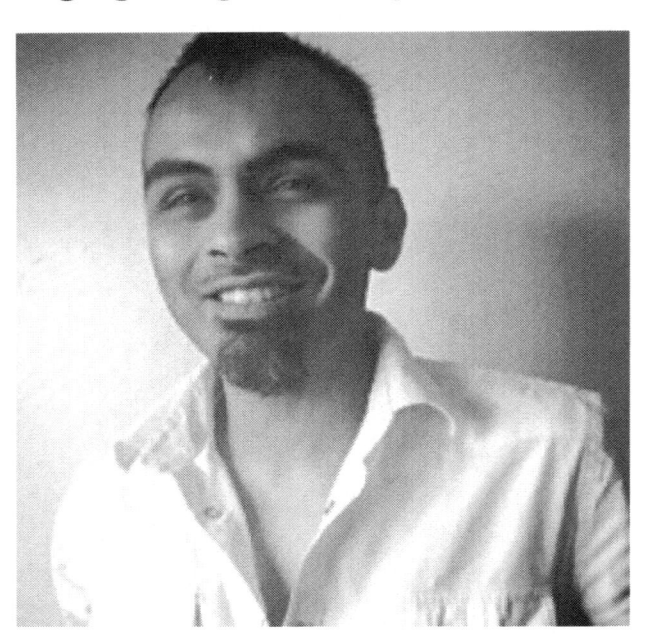

Appendix:
Capoeira Moves and Sequences

Base (Cadeira)

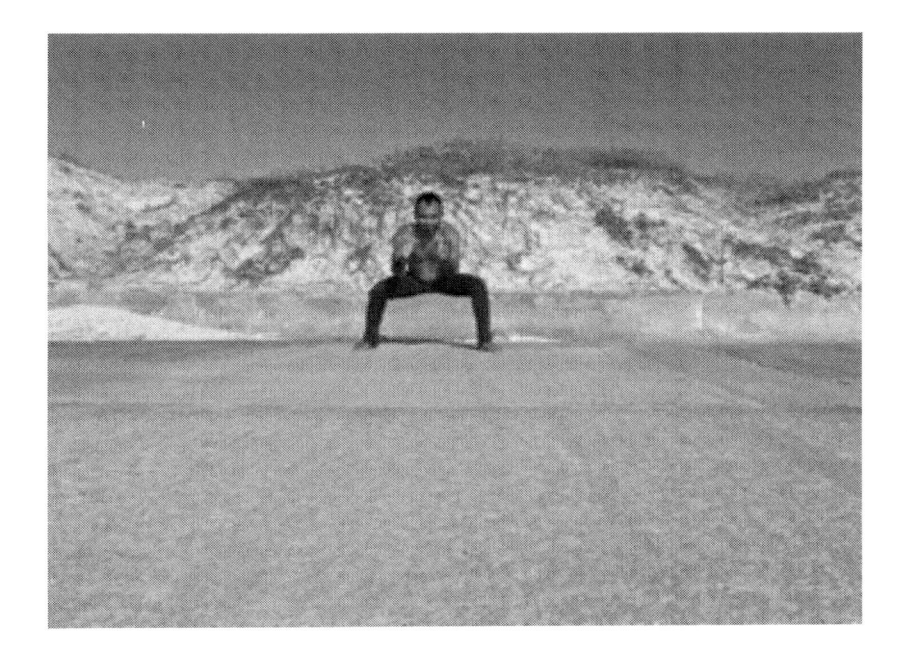

59

Rolé

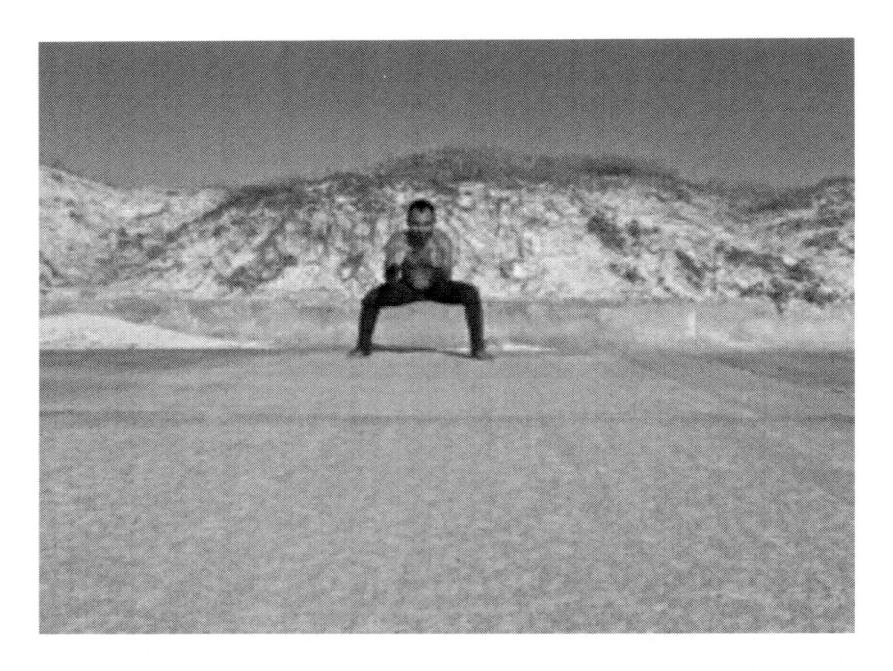

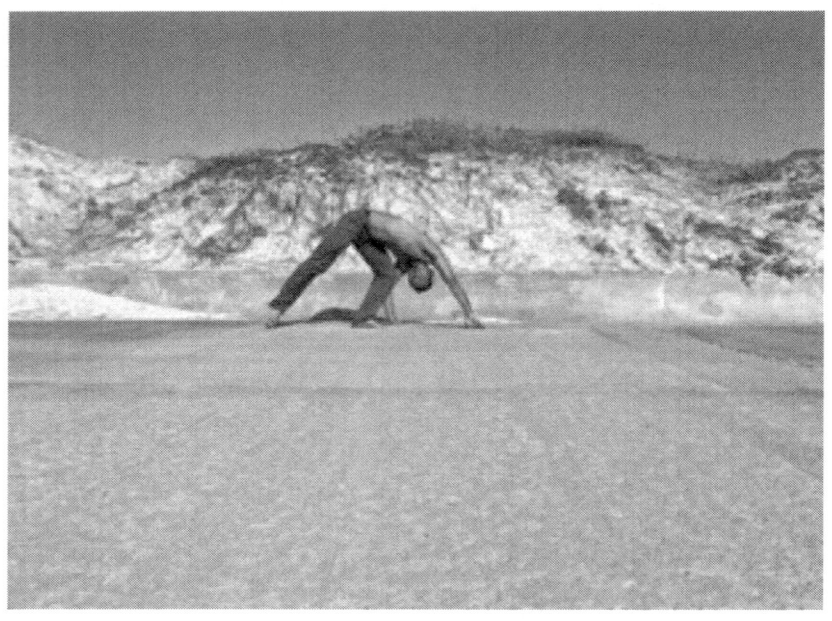

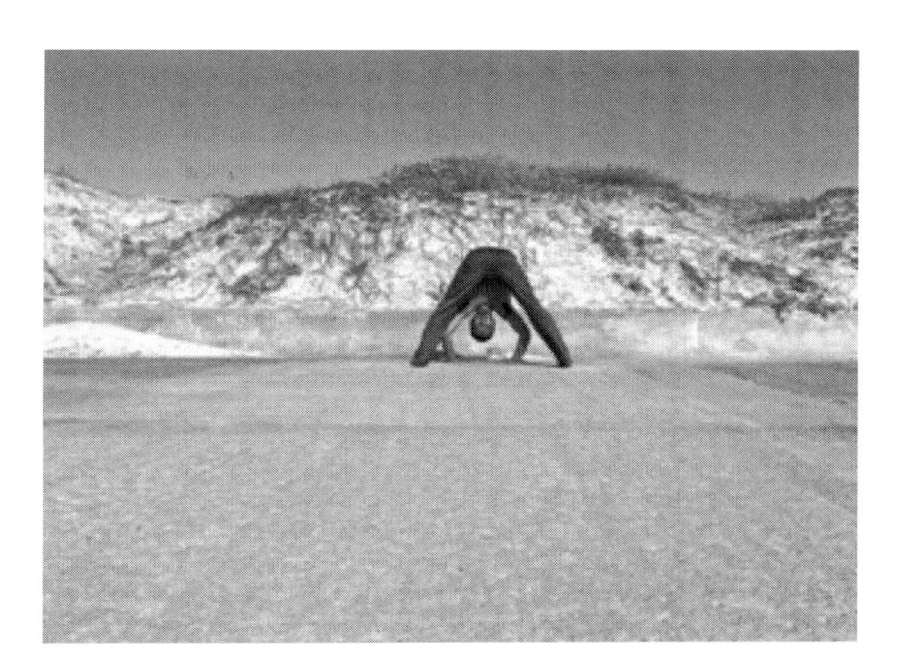

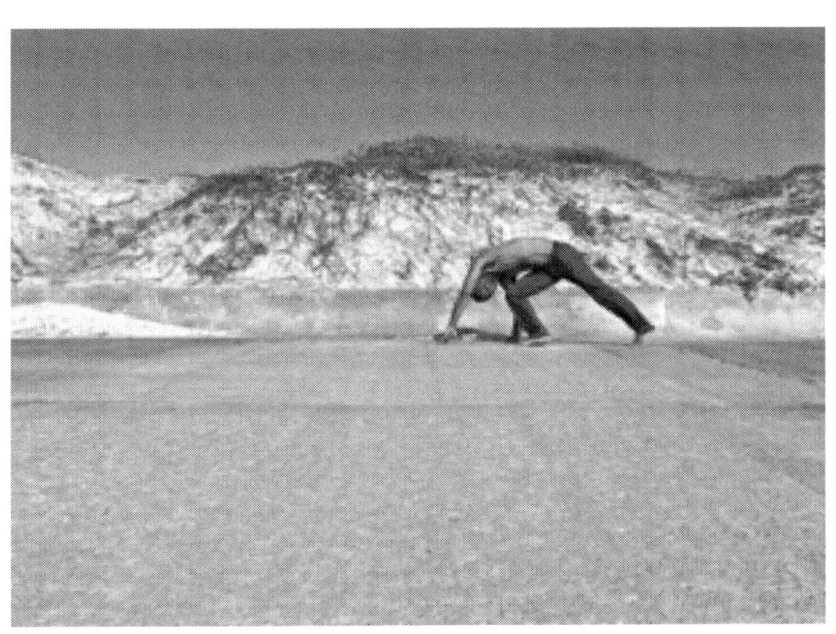

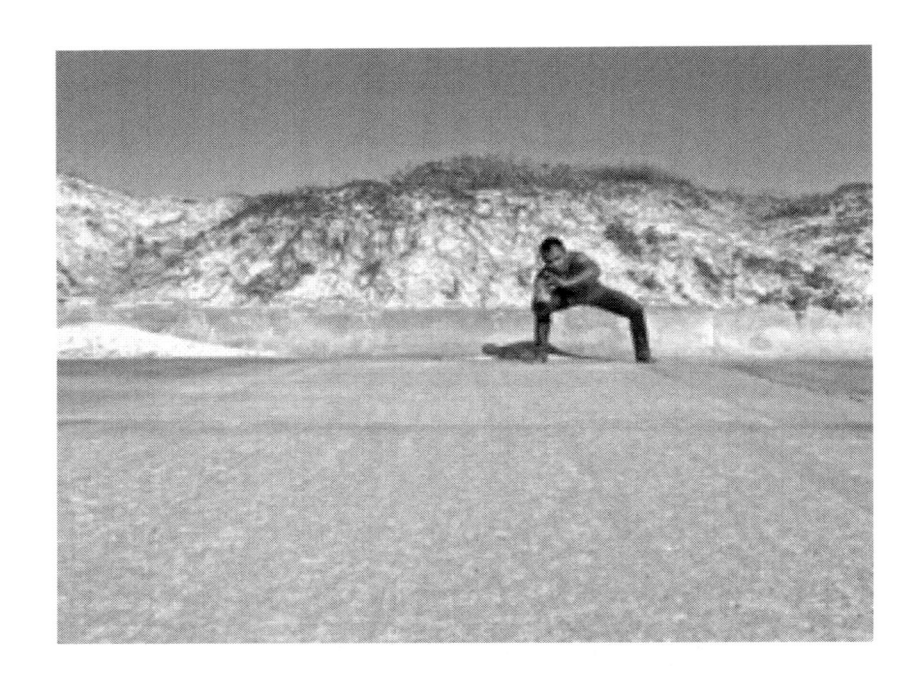

Esquiva

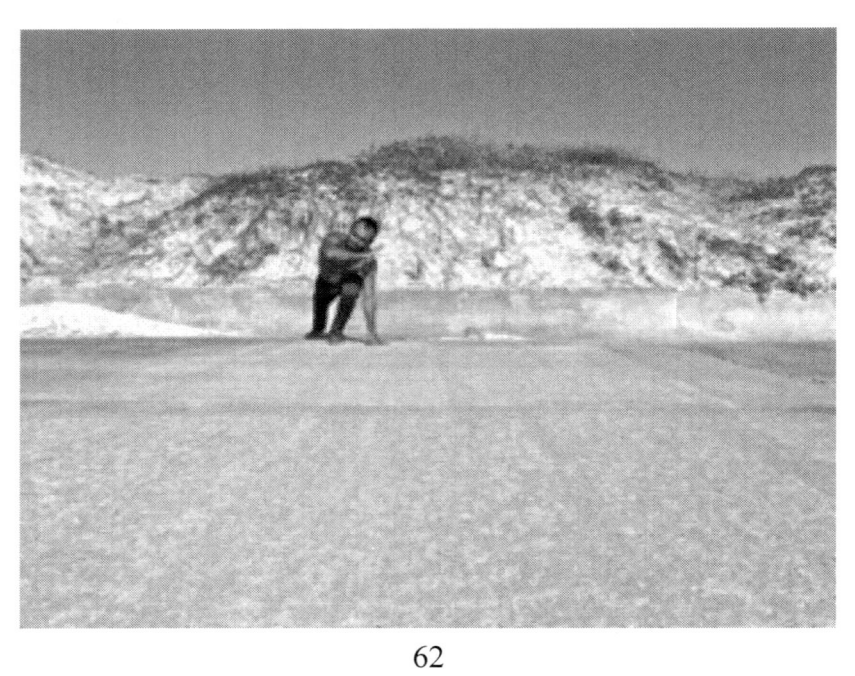

Esquiva Straight to Rolé

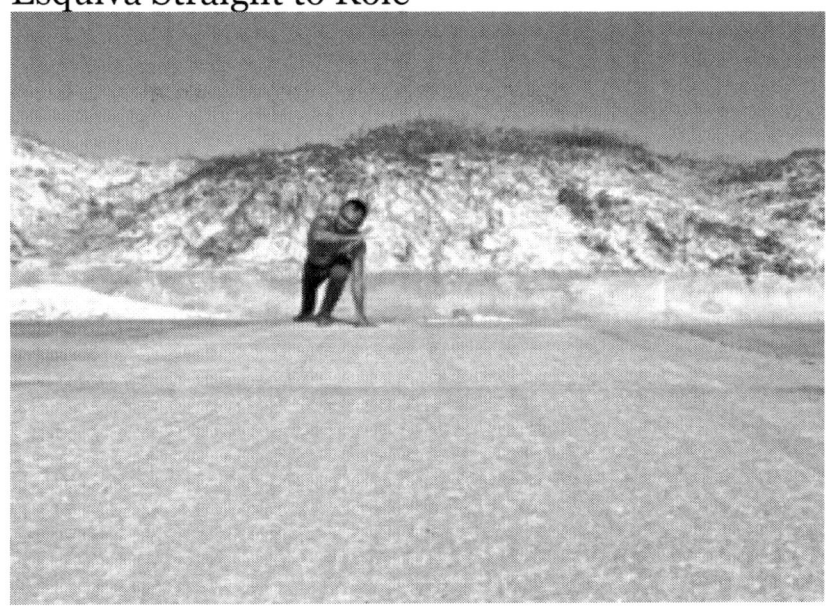

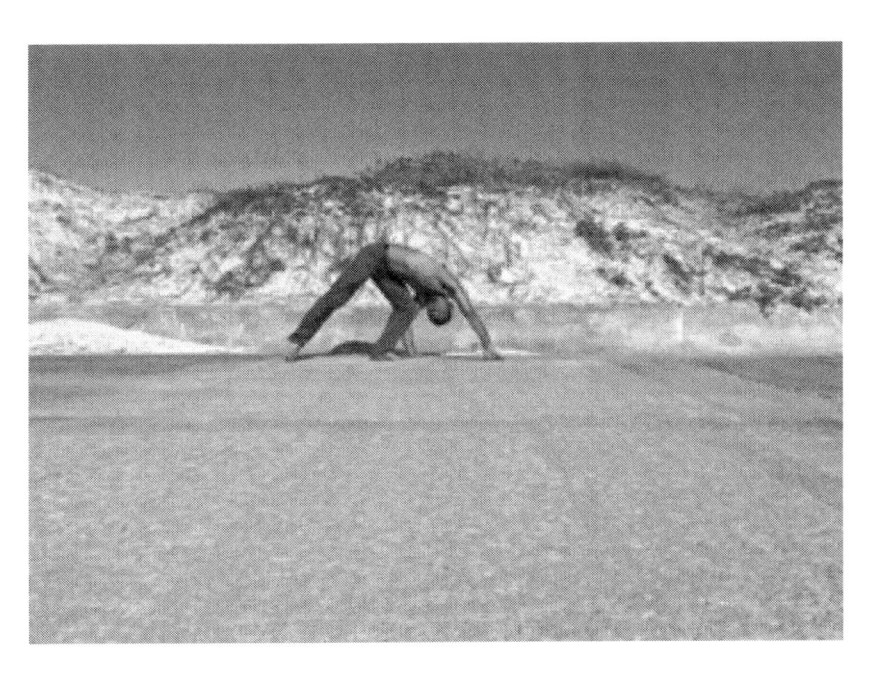

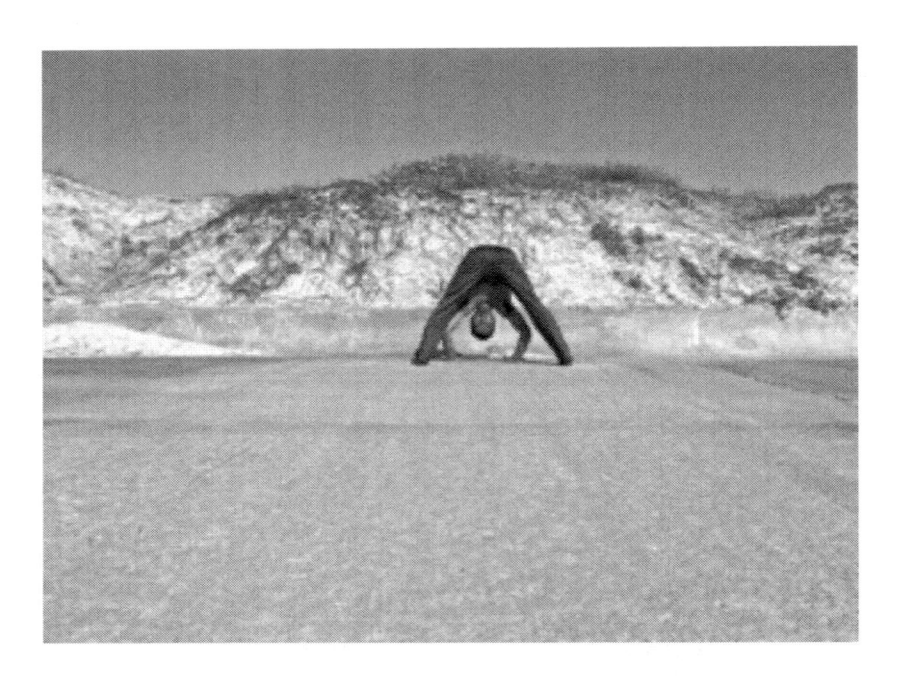

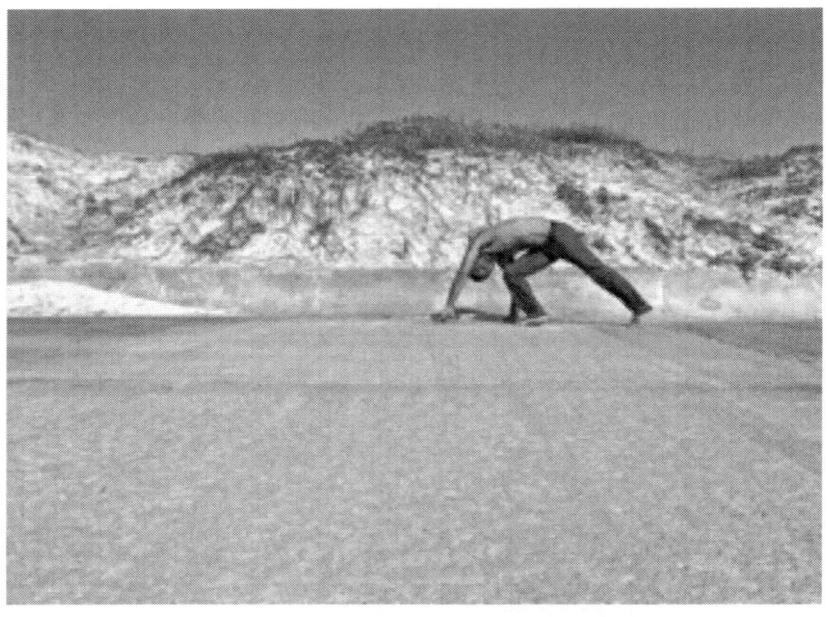

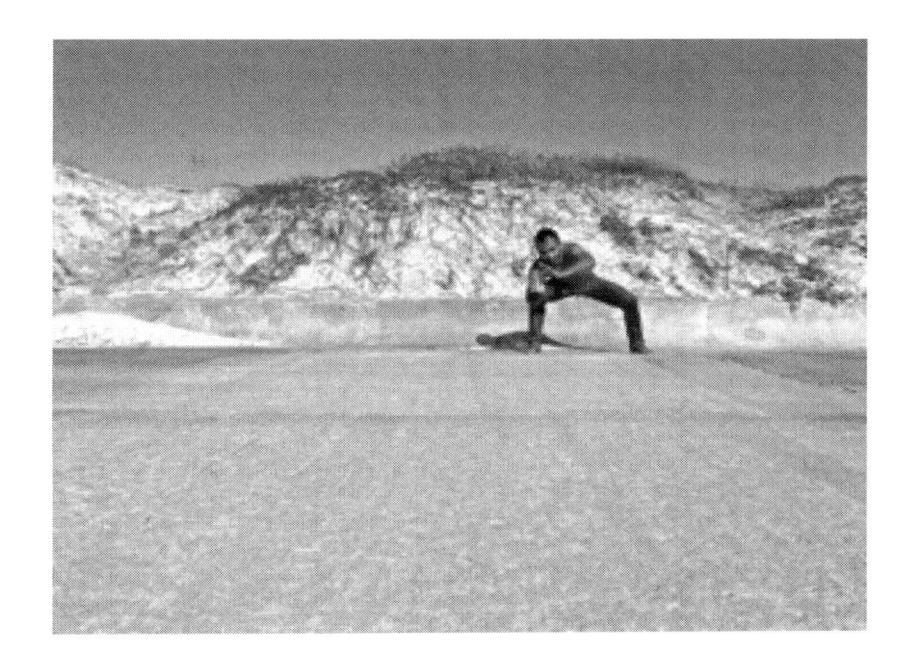

Esquiva Negativa Rolé

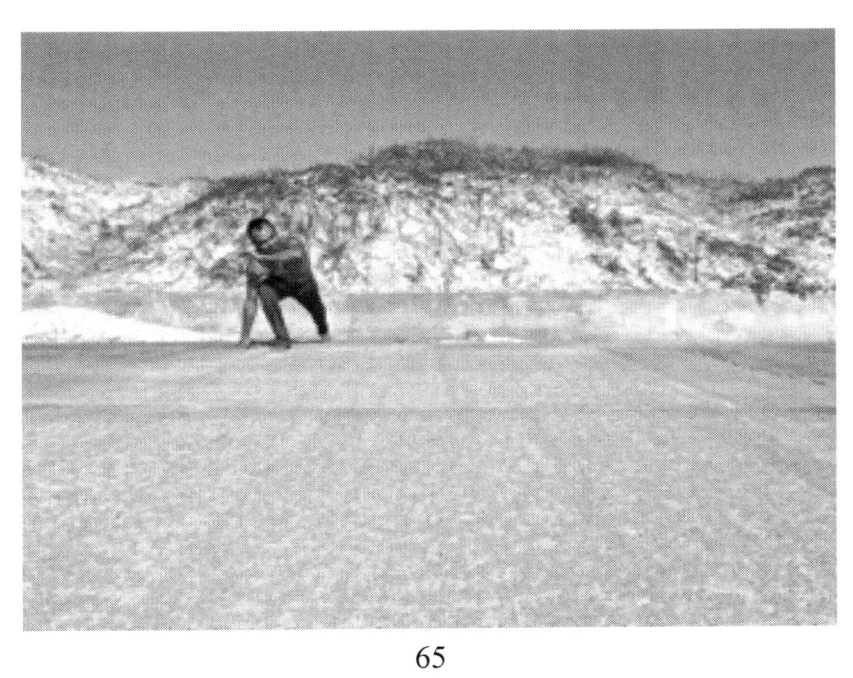

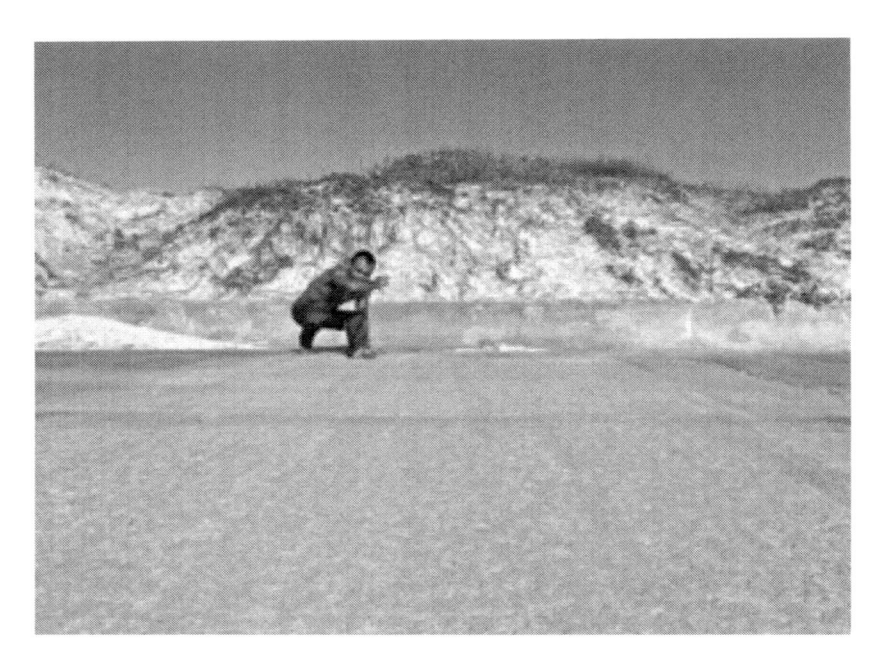

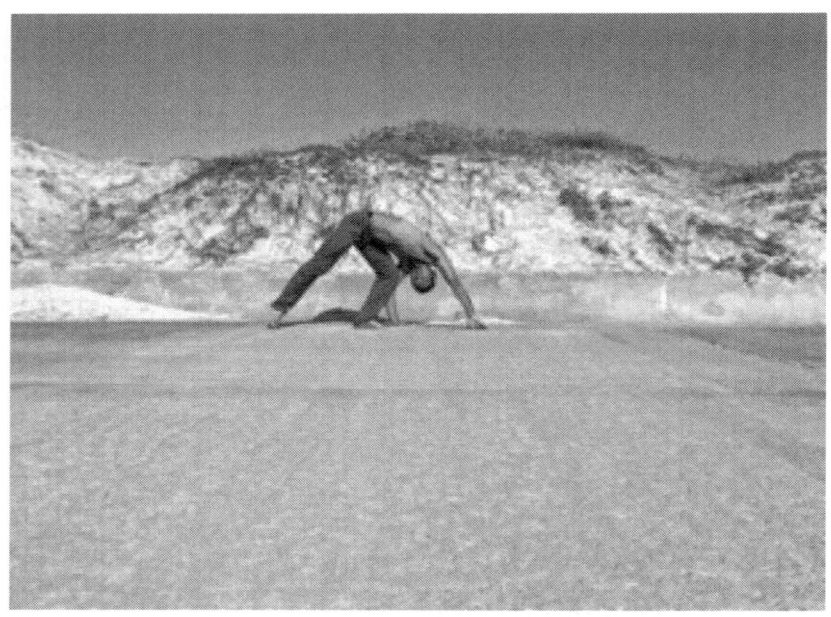

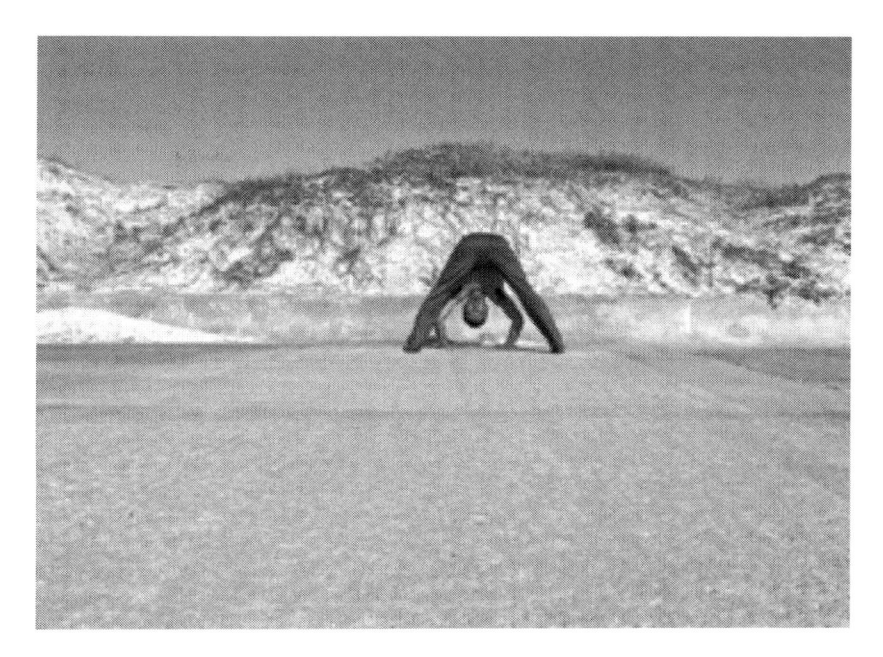

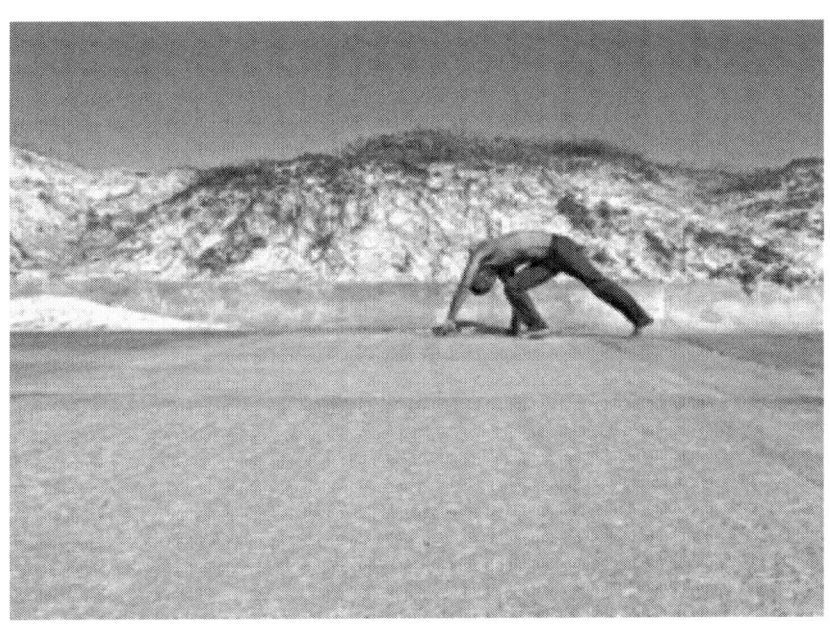

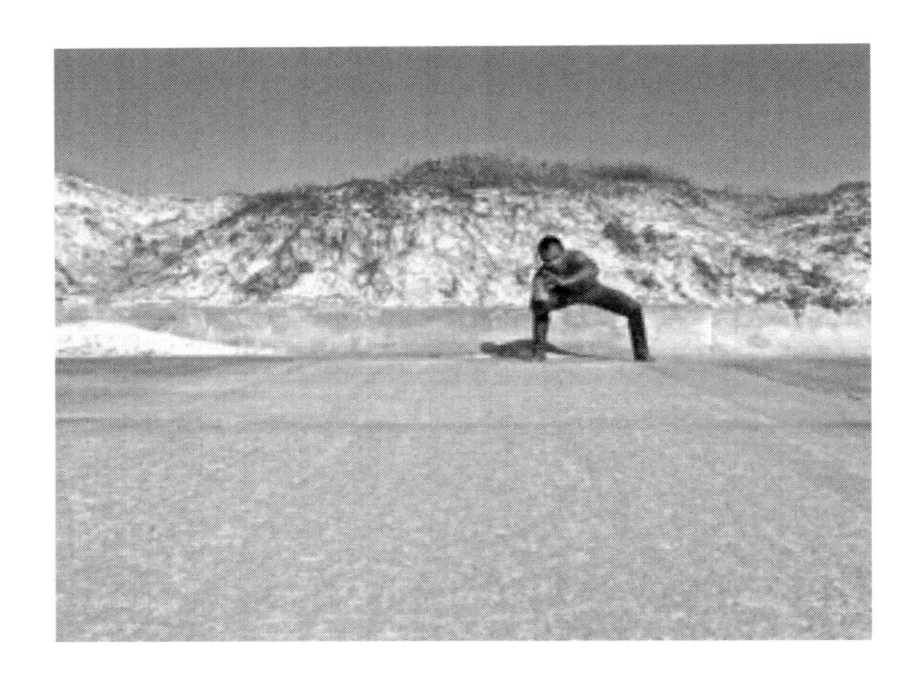

Esquiva Negativa Escapa

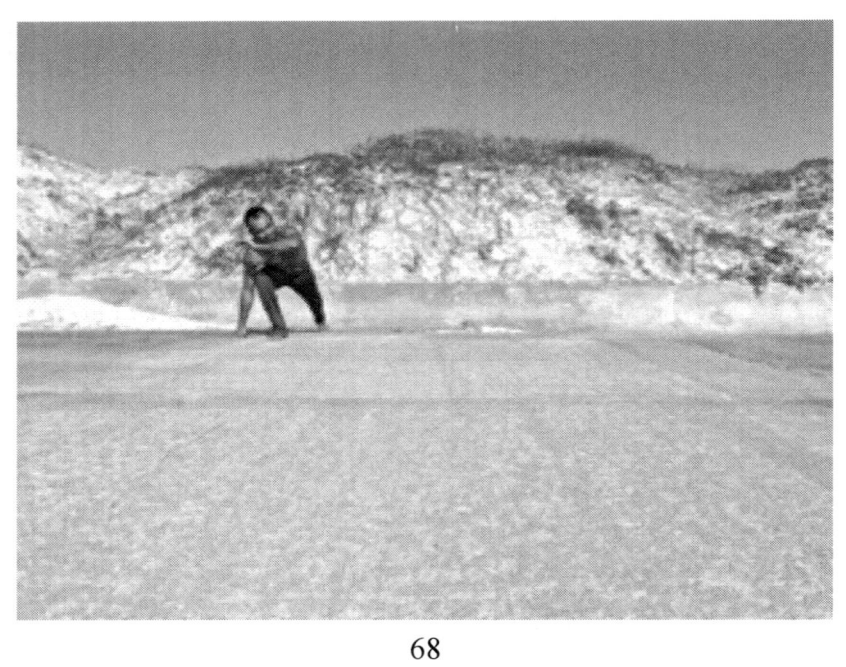

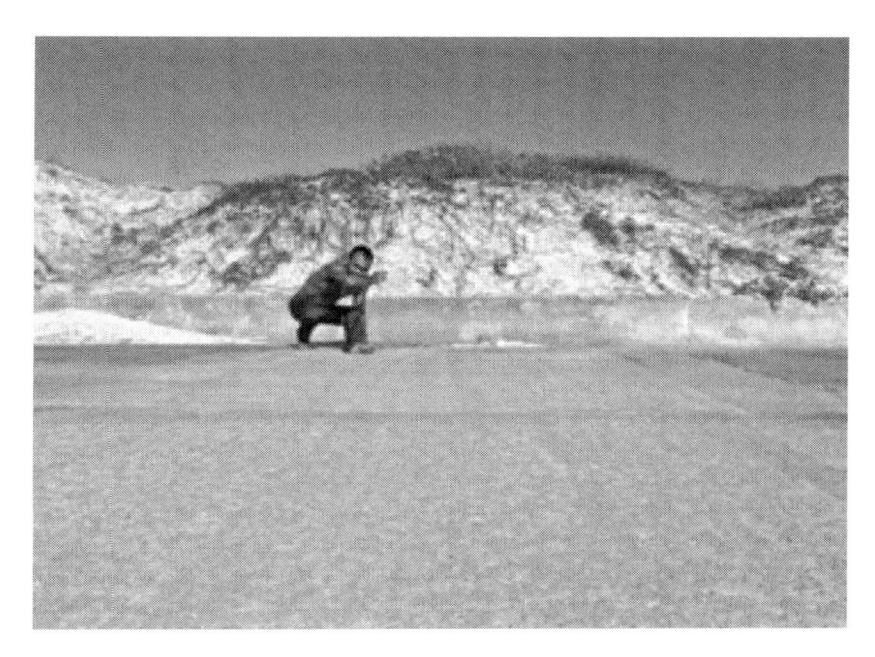

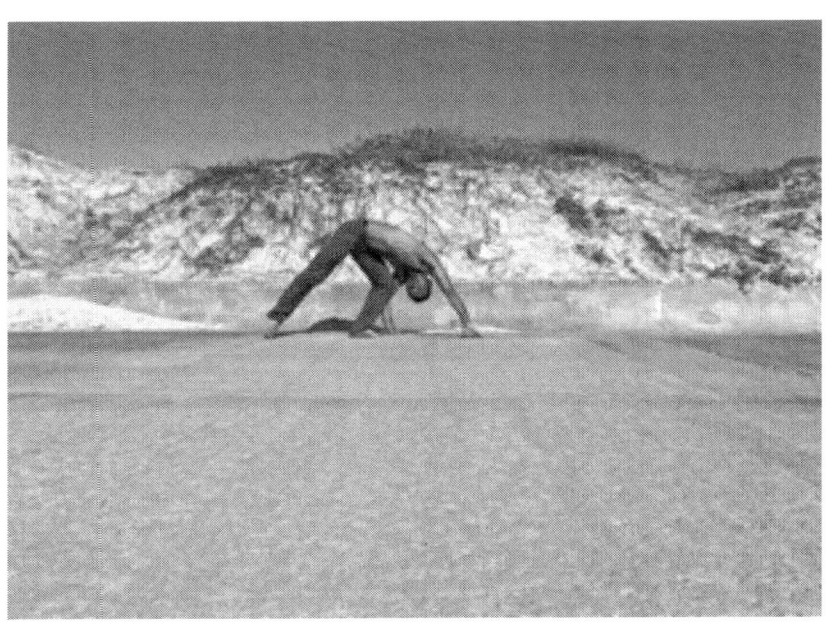

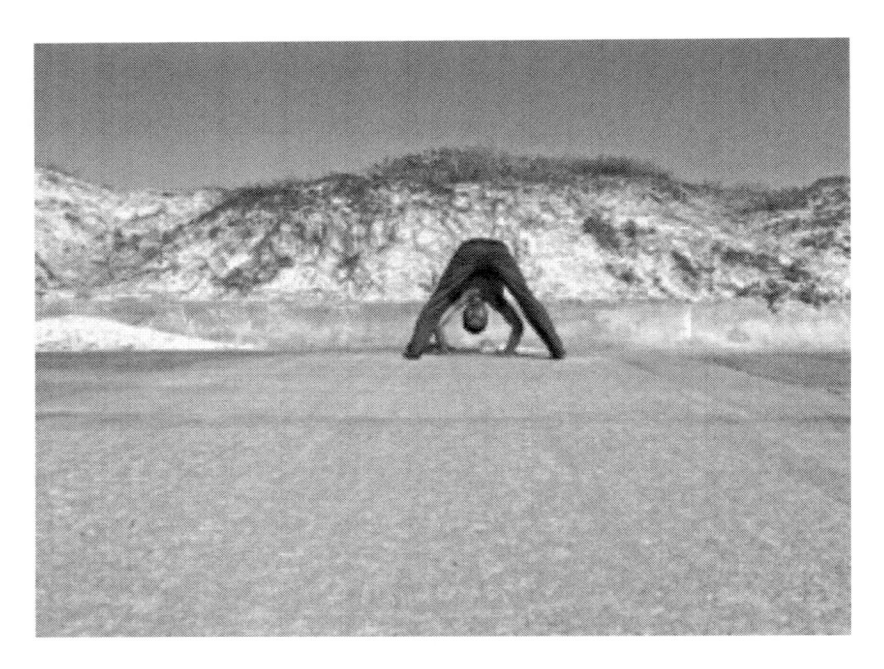

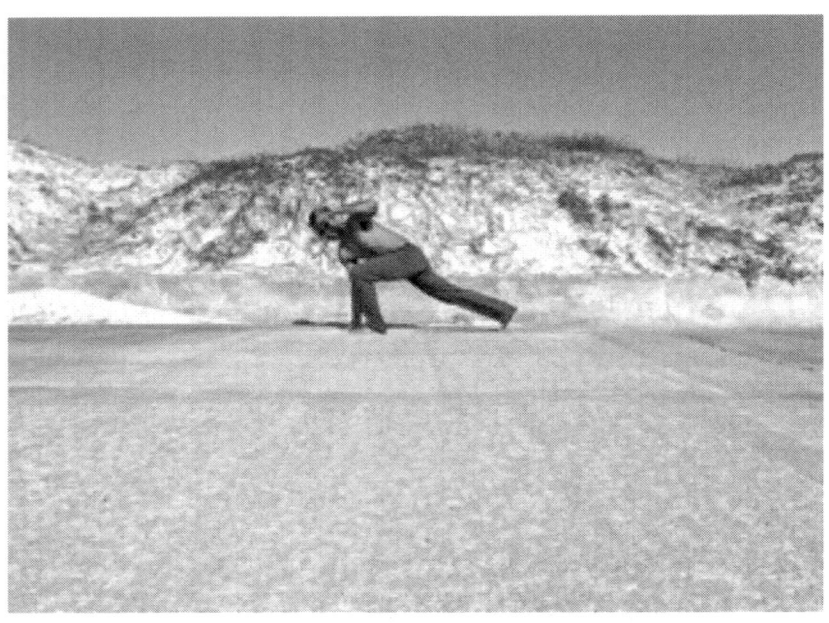

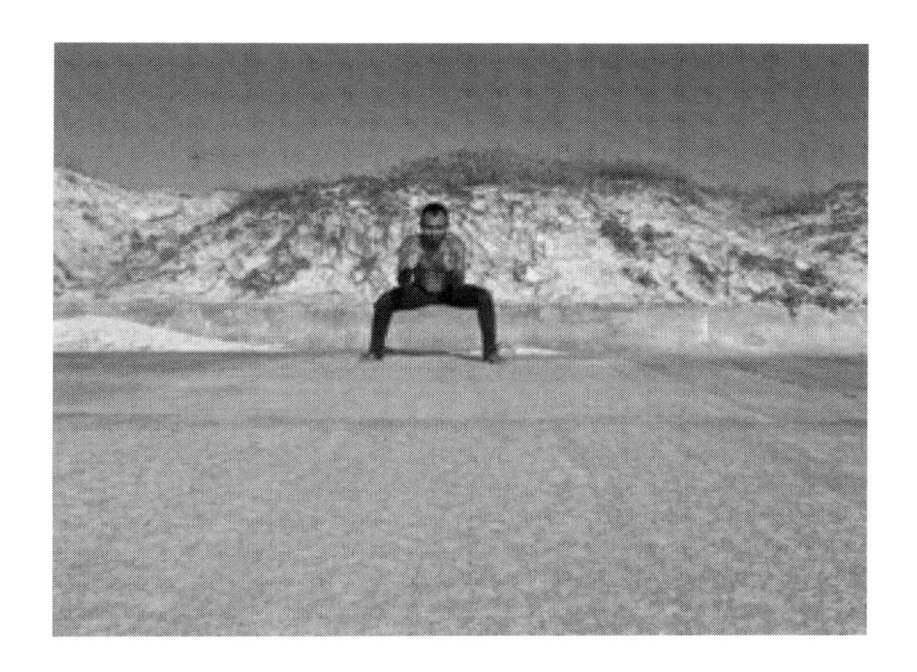

Circular Kicks Land to the Base (Quexada)

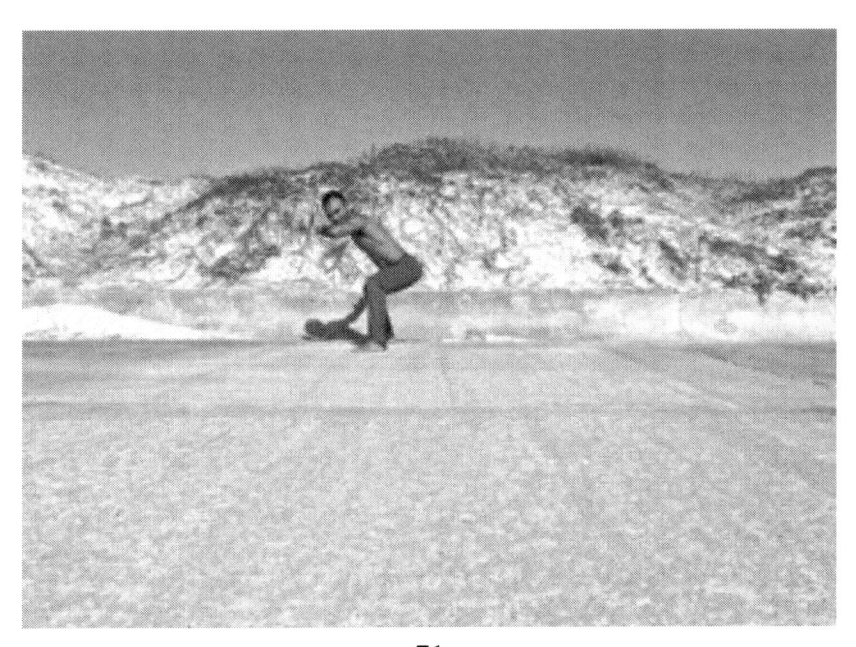

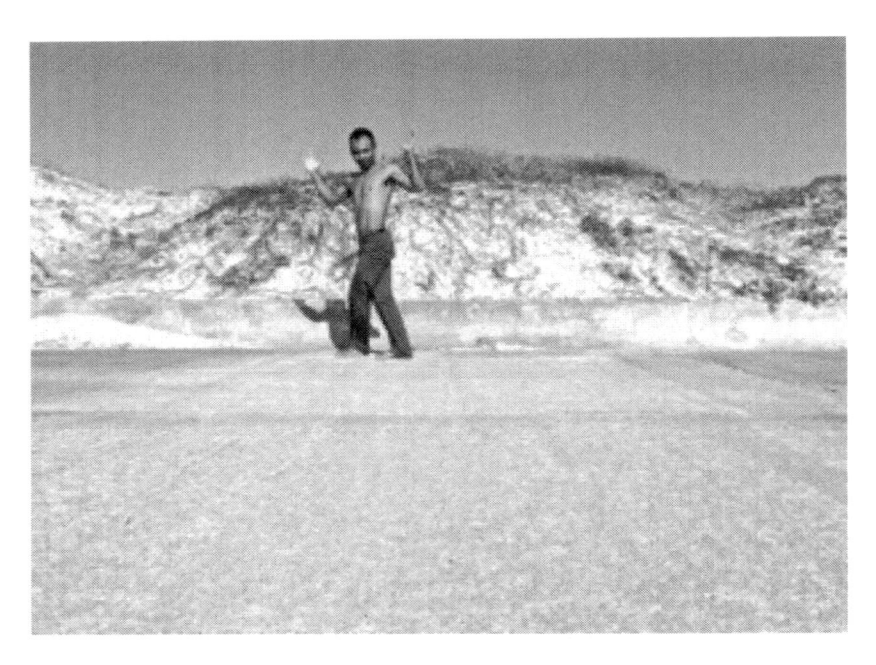

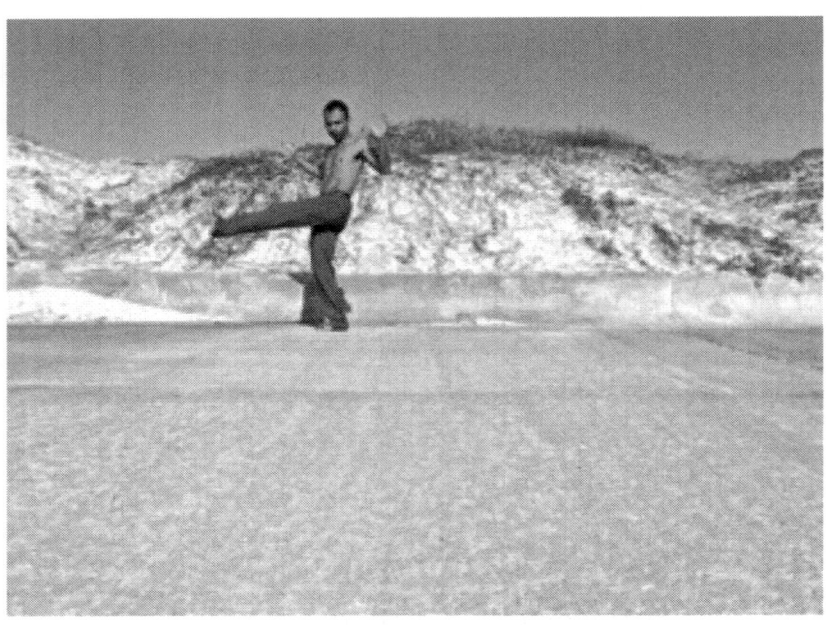

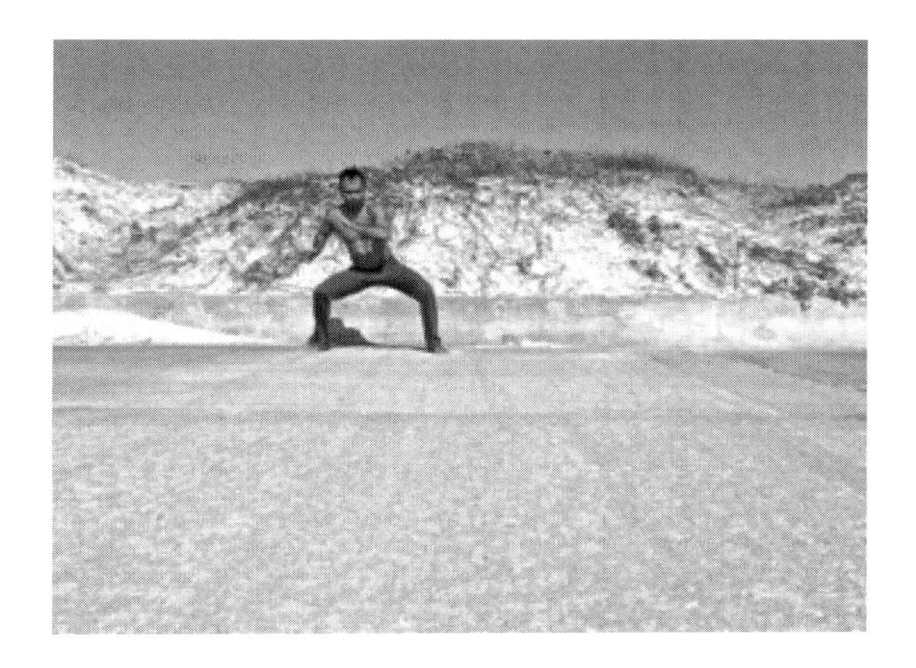

Modifications: Queda de Rins

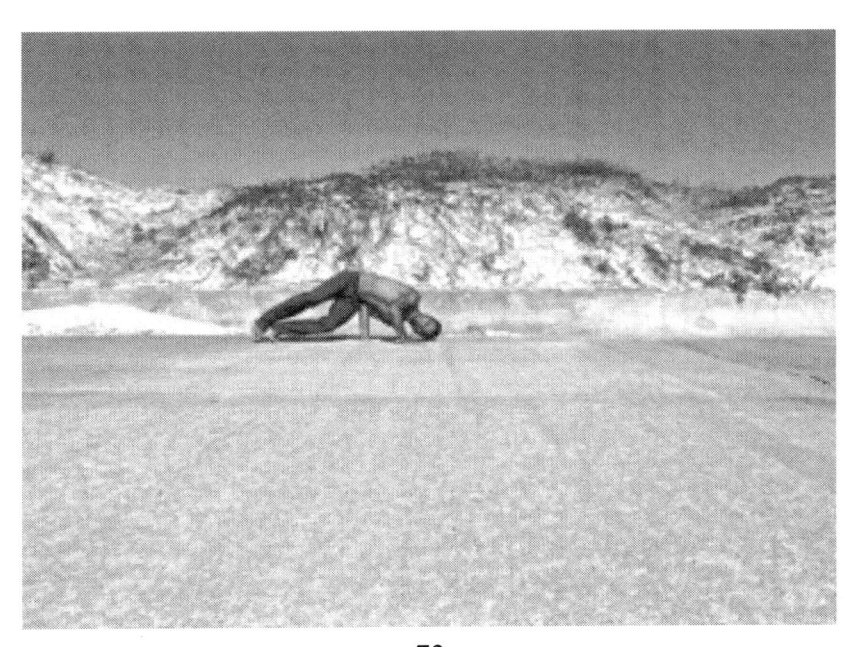

Handstand on Wall

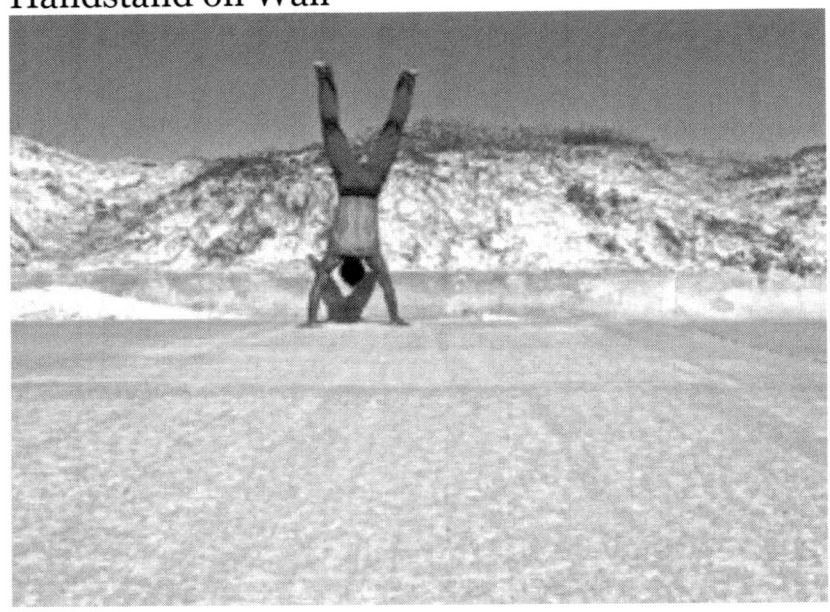

Dismount

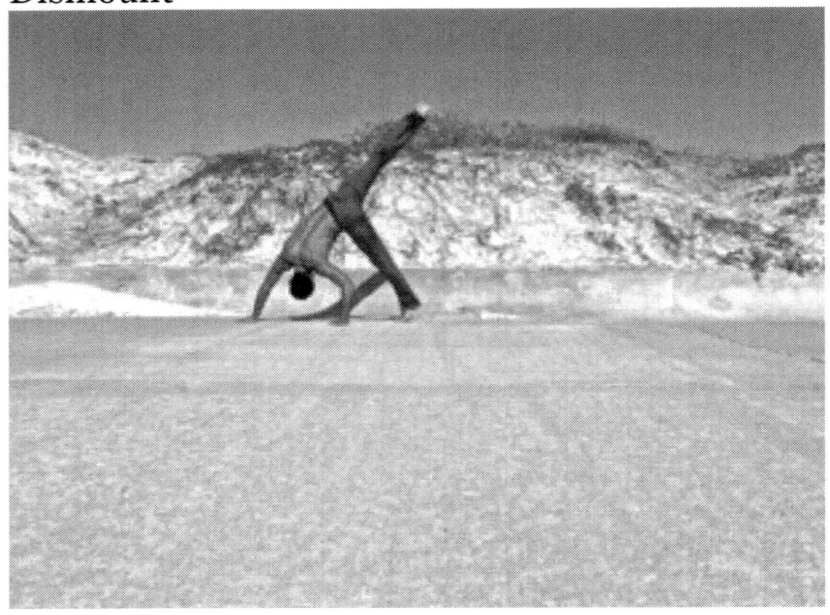

Modifications: Ponte

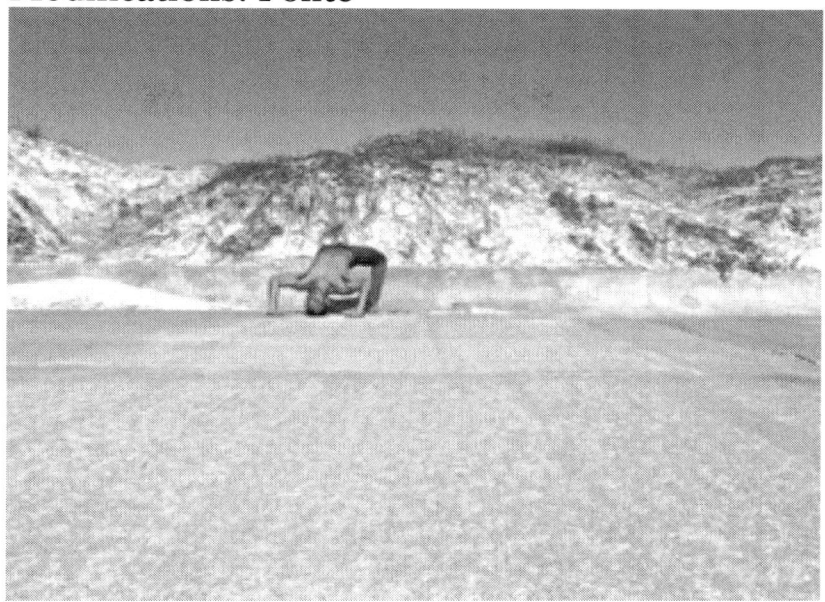

Modifications: Aú (Rolé with a Jump)

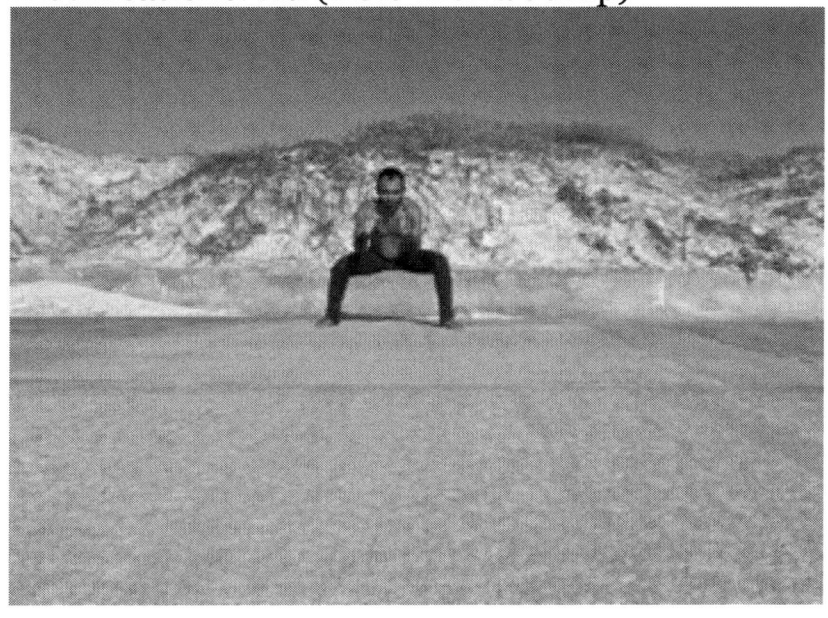

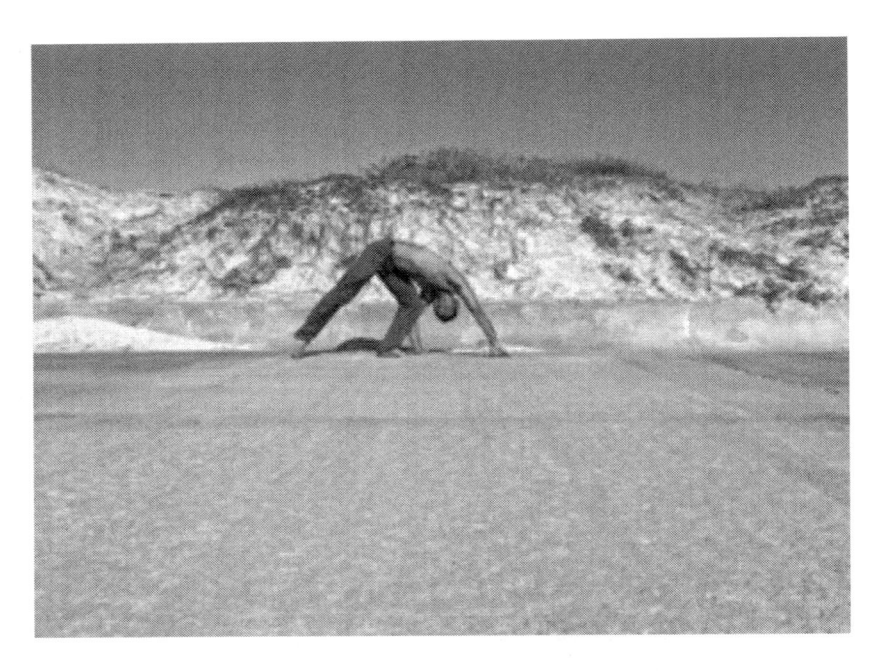

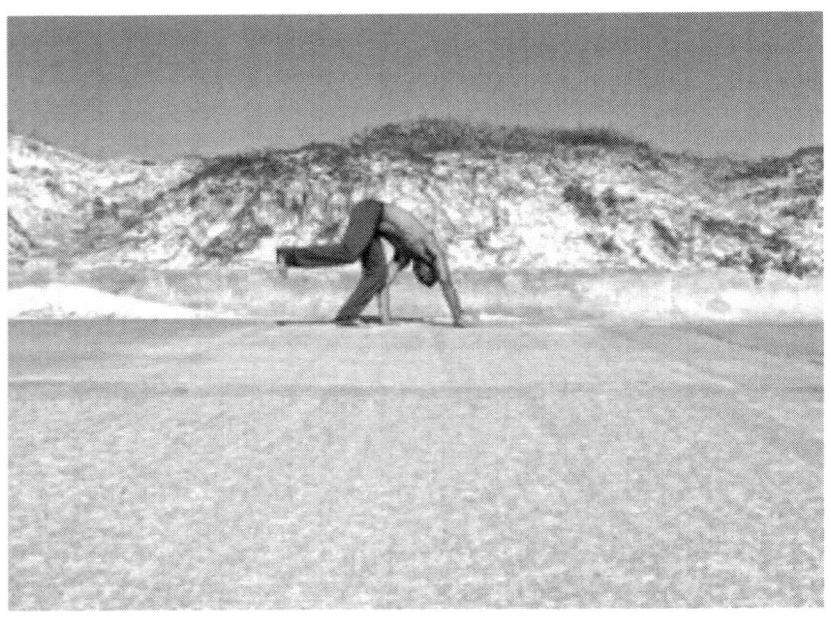

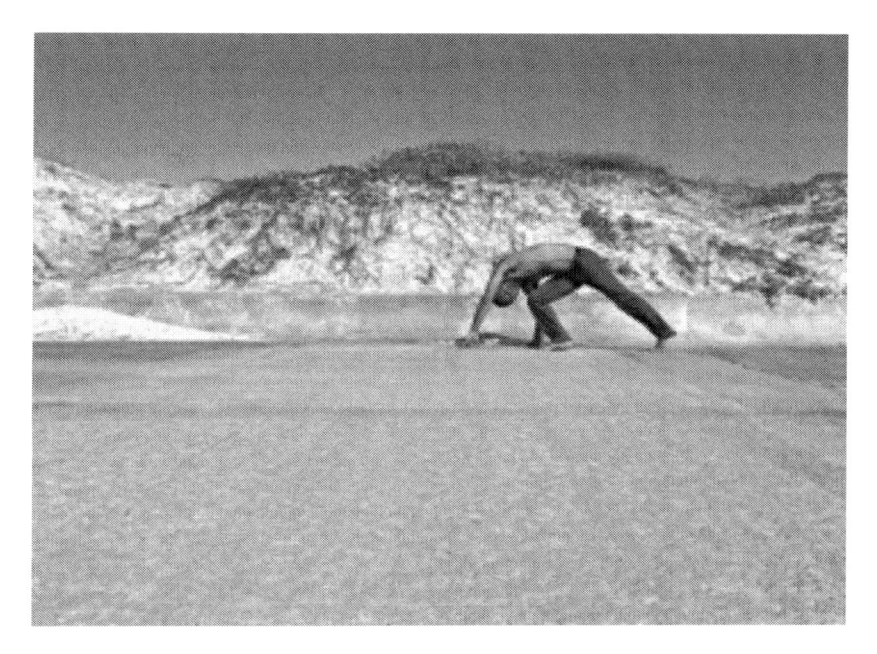

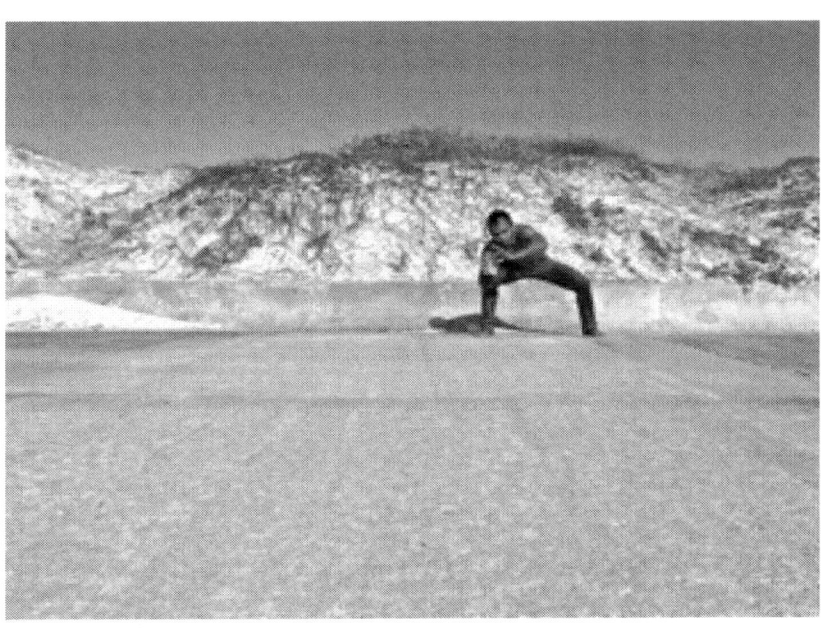

Combinations: Esq. Quebrada Esq. Base

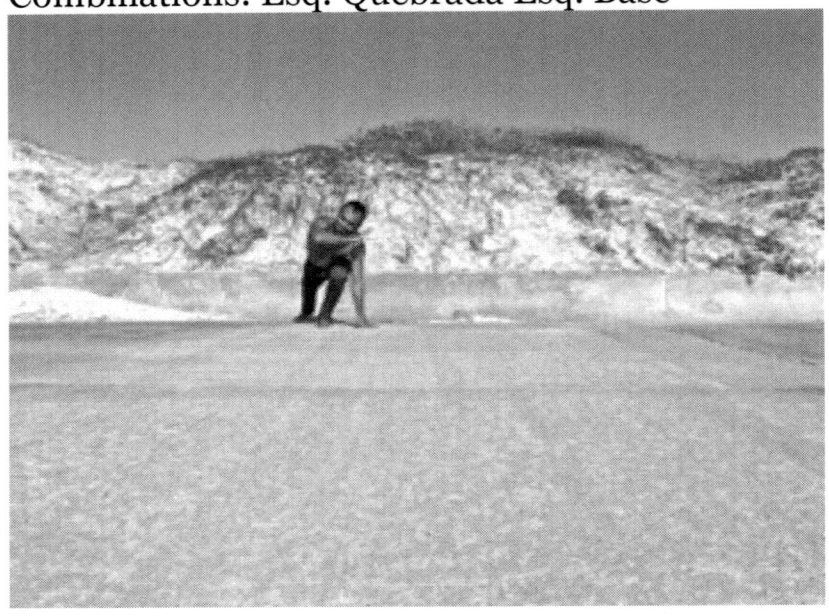

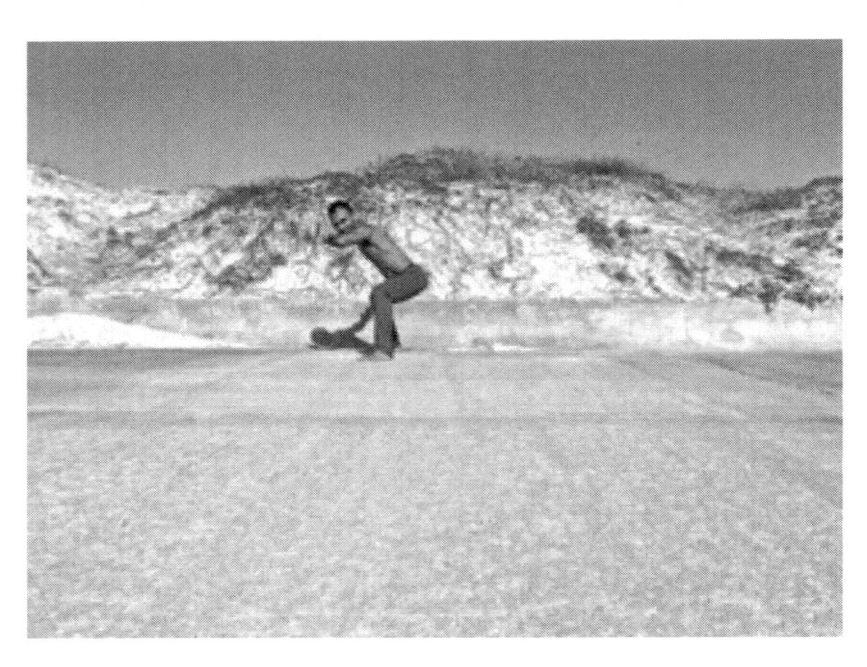

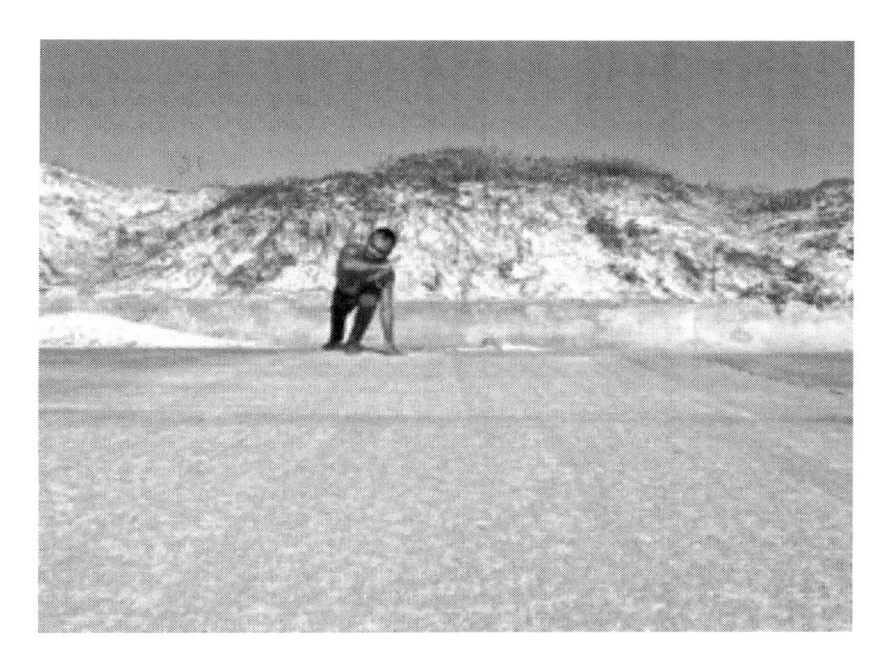

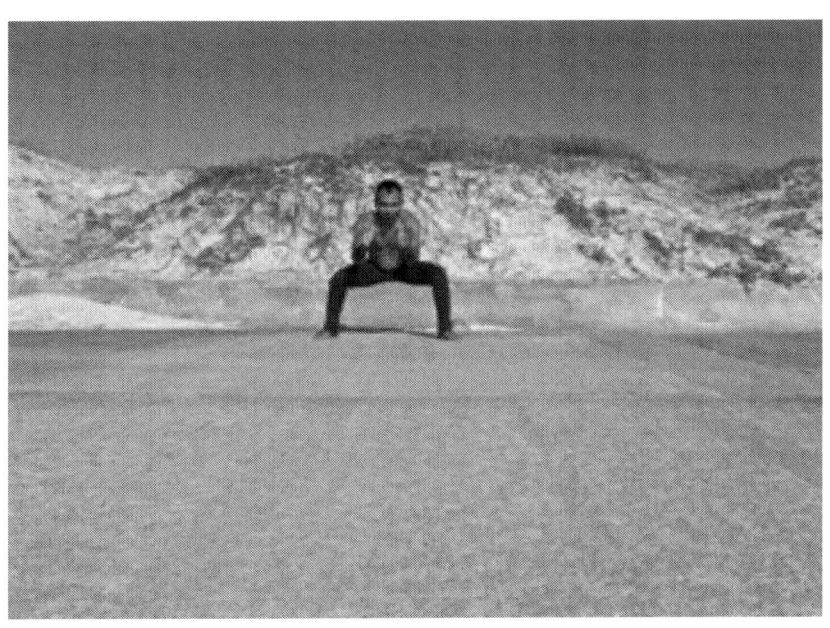

Combinations: Esq. Lat. Left, Right, Left

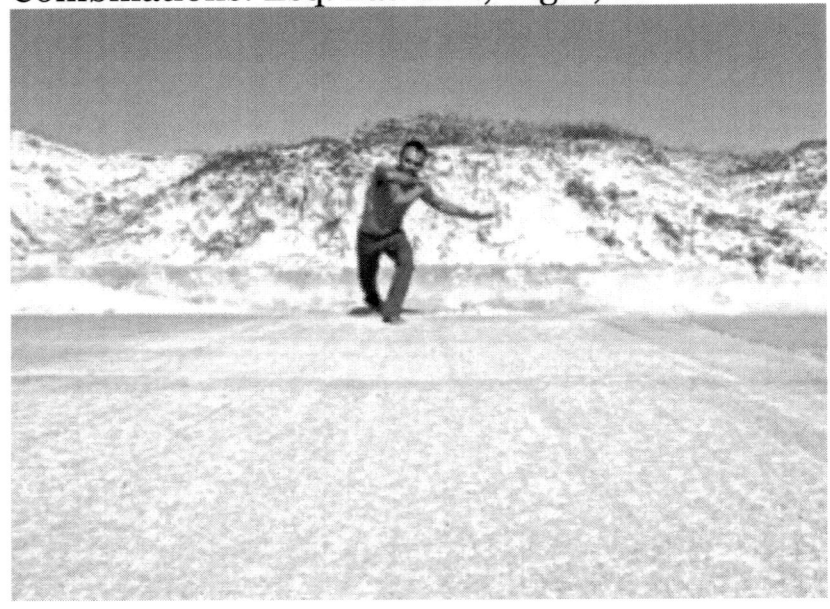

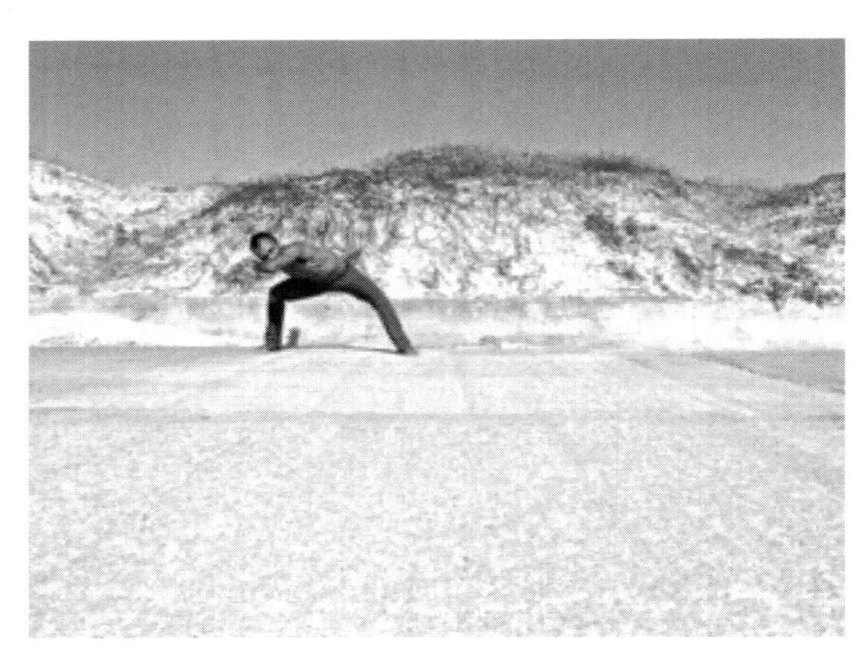

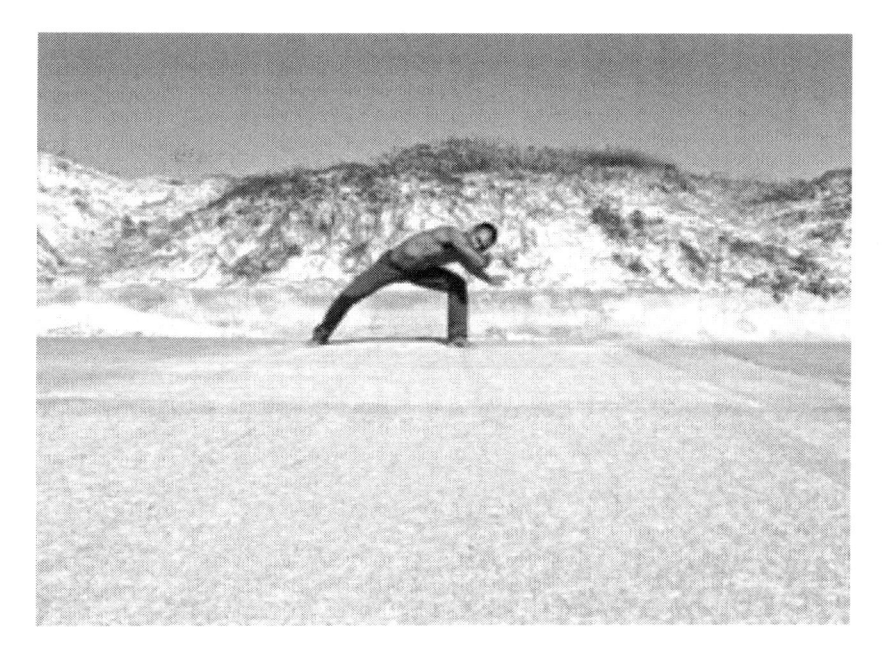

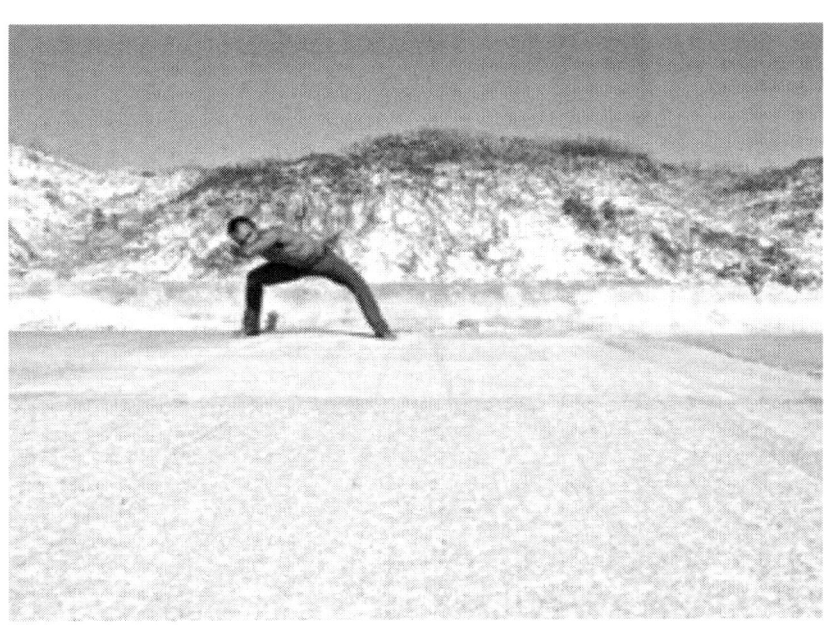

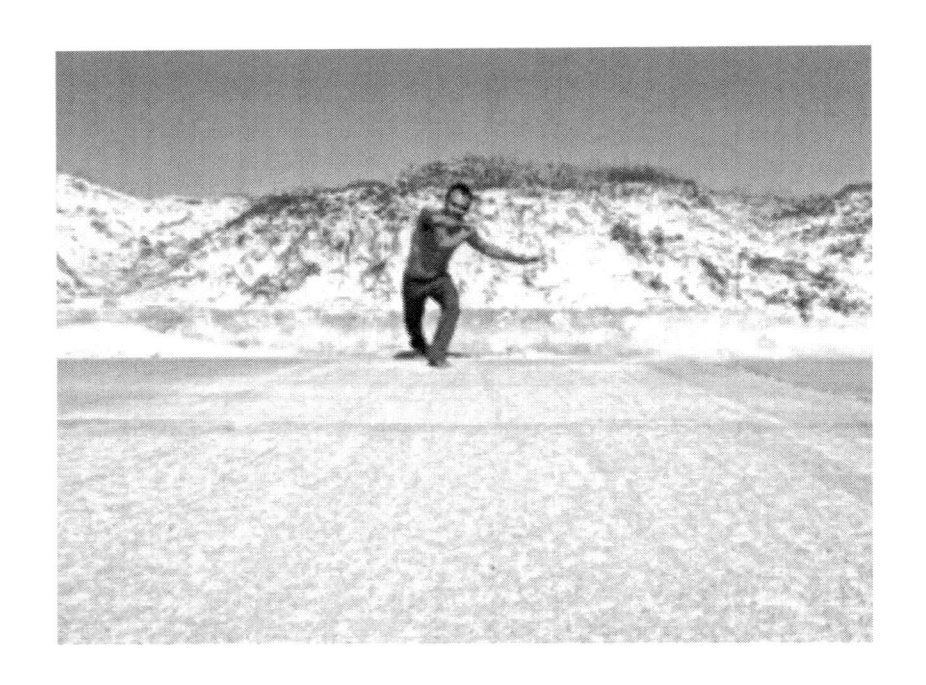

Combinations: Fake MLC, Escapa Look L, R.

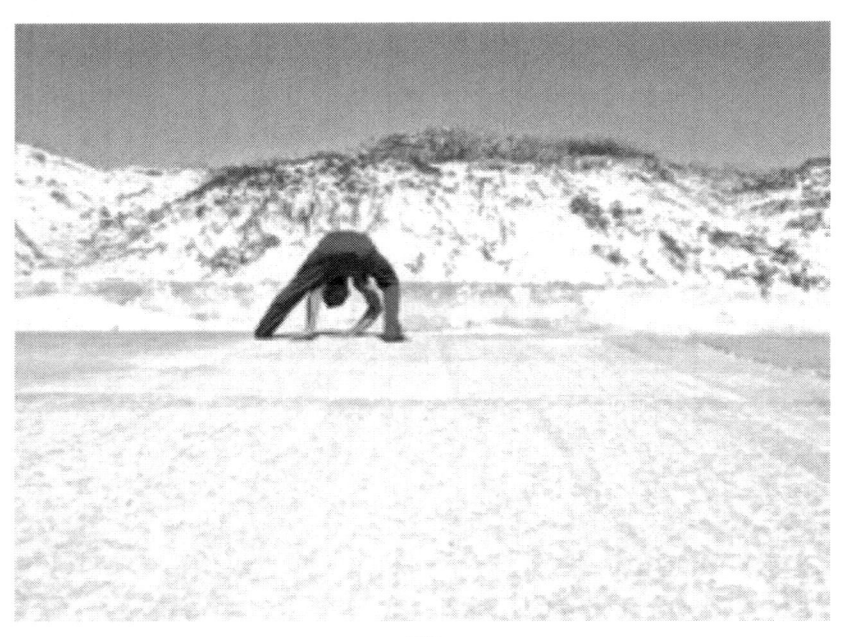

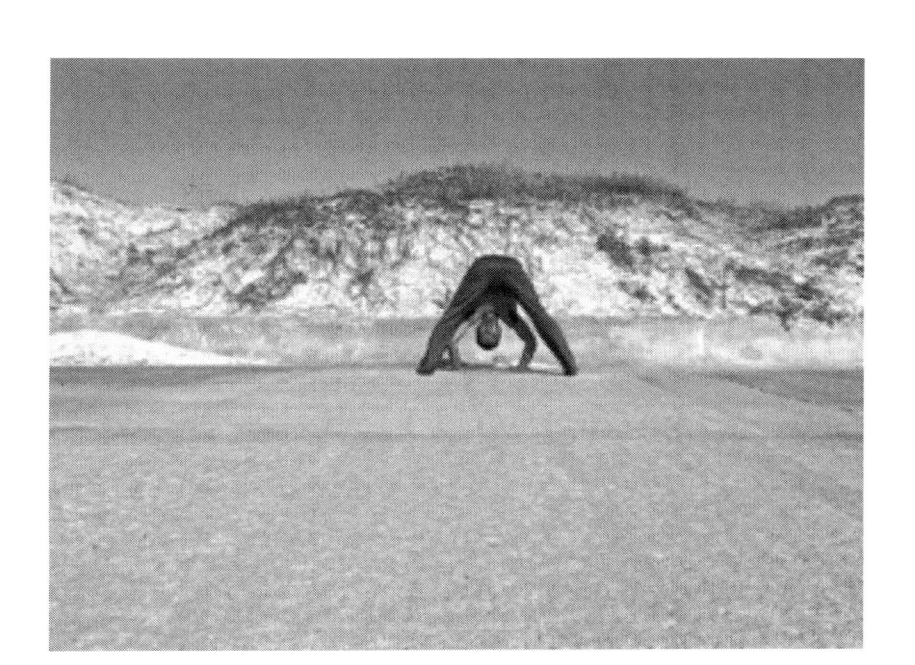

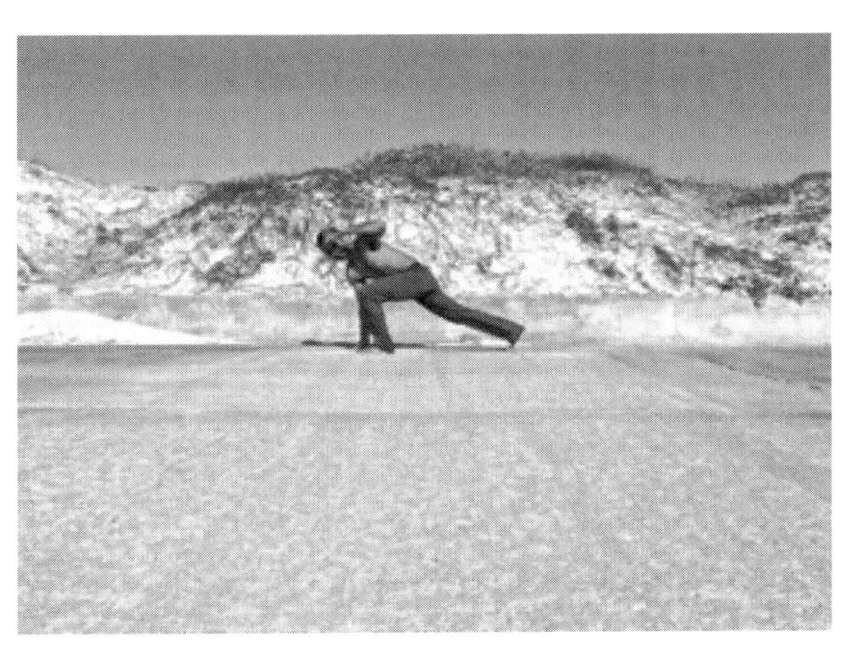

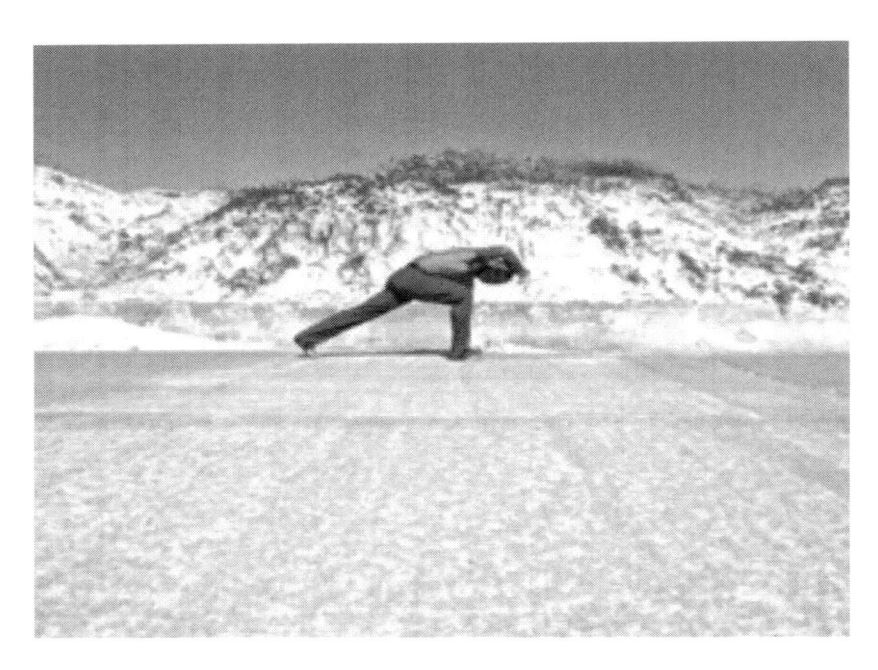

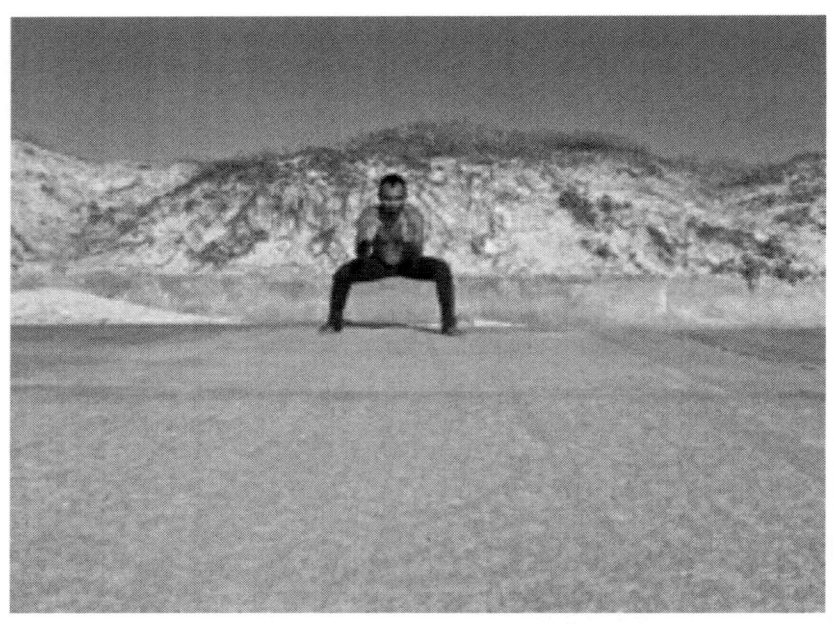

Partner Training: Benção Drill

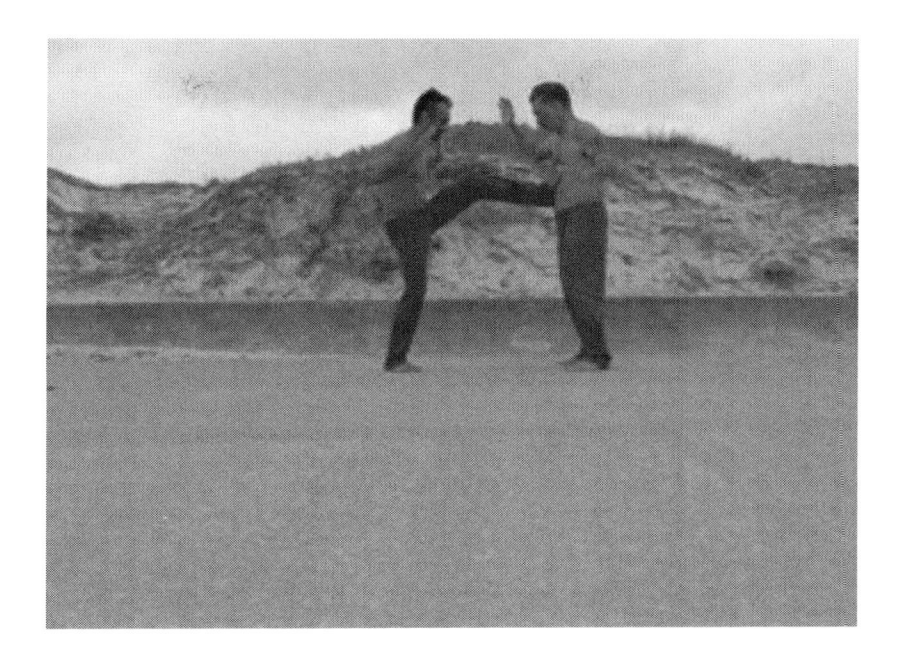

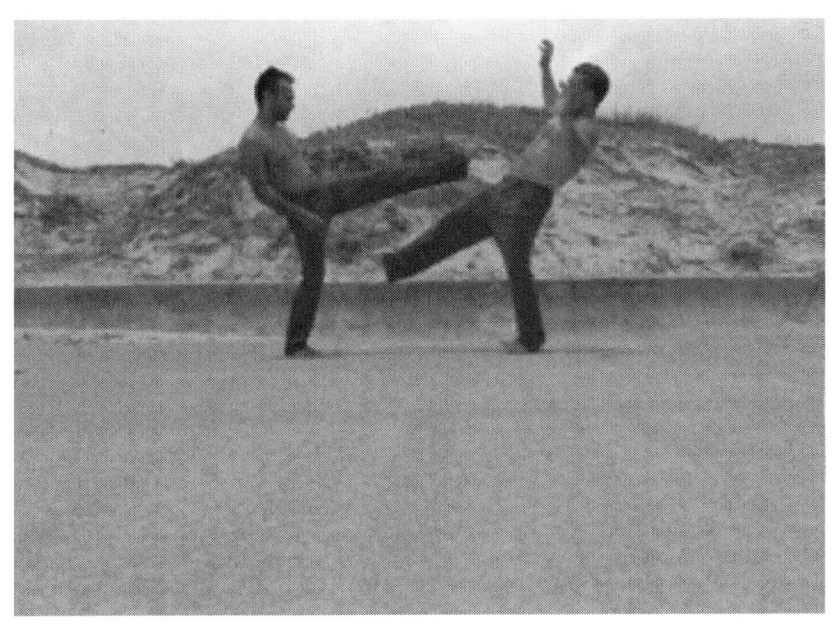

Bonus Chapter:
Capoeira Over 40: Brazil Training Trip

While editing and finalizing this book, I took my first trip to Brazil. You can read all about it on my blog very soon at www.gingaandgrowstrong.com. This was a training and vacationing trip. As an older guy, I knew my training hard would be limited.

Don't get me wrong, I am the king of kicks and long 3 hour training sessions. There was a time when I would wake up every week day at 6 am, and do 1, 000 kicks in my garage. I would go to work and then train Capoeira at my instructors studio. Not enough? Many times I would warm up briefly before class started with 300 kicks while all the other students were messing around waiting for class to start.

As of now, I have been training over 11 years, so I know age does to a body over time. I have many students over 40, and some over 50. This trip was not going to be like the stories I heard in my younger days as a student. I would hear that students would haul off to Brazil in a group of about 10, cram in one of the Mestres' houses sleeping on the floor, and train 3 times a day.

Many times students would get sick, because of overtraining, no clean water, and lack of proper nourishment. Awesome, right? Well, as much as this appealed to me in my younger years, times have changed. Technology has changed as well. Airbnb did not exist back then nor Uber. These two applications in itself made my trip way different than it would've 10 years ago.

There were stories of brutal rodas, bad travel arrangements, and muggings. No thanks! I thought this material was relevant to this book since I am older, and modified our trip for an older Capoeira.

As mentioned earlier, I have documented the whole trip in my journal and took good video documentation that will make its way on my blog real soon. But here's the trip as what it relates to Capoeira Over 40.

This trip was organized at least 6 months in advanced, so we had sufficient time to prepare ho we would pack, how much we would train, and add in any other tourist destinations and activities. The plan was to travel in a small group of 4 so we can rent a car and split the cost.

We would split the cost of hotels, Airbnb houses, Ubers, taxis, and any other big expenses. As it turned out, one of our party got held up in customs in São Paulo for not having his visa, so it turned out to be just the 3 of us: Mestrando Advogado, Graduado O Rei, and Aluno Olho de Tigre.

We would be staying for 2 1/2 weeks and travel throughout 4 states, Rio de Janeiro, Minas Gerais, Bahia, and Espirito Santo. We would train for 4 days in the first week, saving the other 3 days for travel and leisure.

The second week we would train 3 days and save the other 4 days for travel and leisure. The remaining 3 days were for attending a Capoeira batizado and travel a long, long way back to Rio de Janeiro for our return flight home.

Our training regimen planned was going to be perfect. A lot of classes (once a day) and one or two rodas a week. Sounds like a lot for an old guy, but it really wasn't. Some days there was time for recuperation, and others there was less, however, we only trained once a day unlike the stories of old.

As it turned out, we had several days of tourist activities and fun. Here is the trip on brief play by play description. Base your trip on how you feel physically, and remember you can always rest if you need to. Don't feel pressured to train past your physical limits. The year is 2017, not 1997. You want to represent your country well as a gringo training in Brazil, but safety first.

We arrived in Rio de Janeiro and spent two days of leisure on Copacabana beach and some night life. We then hopped in our rental car for about 6 hours to travel into the interior of Brazil to Belo Horizonte (Minas Gerais). The first day we got there, on a Sunday, we attended a roda at Praça 7 in front of an old church. These guys were awesome. It seemed that the lowest ranking player in attendance was a Professor, however, as the games went on, a couple instrutor level guys trickled in.

We set up training for nightly class with Grão Mestre Dunga for all week. Everyday we trained at 7 pm, and during the day we took private percussion lessons, dance lessons, and toured around the city. On Thursday they had a roda where a bunch of big shots attended and gave us the Brazilian hospitality.

Everyone was really respectful and happy to help us learn their Capoeira culture. This is not always the case. Make sure you know who you're training with and if they accept foreigners training Capoeira. Many believe that gringos shouldn't training or teaching Capoeira. Be careful.

We traveled from Belo Horizonte the next day, Friday, to Porto Seguro (Bahia). This was one of the worst days of traveling of the whole trip (13 hours). When we arrived, we did not have access to our room we paid for on Airbnb. You can read about the whole story on my blog. We spent the next 3 days in beach paradise before departing on Monday to Espirito Santo.

We had a lot of time to recover from the long drive and embarked on another long drive to Conçeição da Barra. Here, we relaxed the first night and then while waiting for our Capoeira connection to come through didn't end up training until Wednesday. So we took the liberty of going to the beach, taking a buggy tour, and enjoying the small beach town's sights.

Class and roda on Wednesday, Berimbau making workshop on Thursday, Friday night roda with about 60 capoeiristas, and then a batizado on Saturday. Of course, there were after parties, and churrascos, so the day was filled with amazing Brazilian energy!

Our bodies were sore from training, but again, we took ample time to recover the next days. There was a lot of down time and relaxing going on during the day. The Sunday was reserved for our long 9 hour drive back to Rio. We stumbled into our hotel room and melted into the bed. In the morning we took the shuttle to the airport for our long flights home.

This is just my journey. Depending on your physical and financial means, yours will differ. If you can't afford or don't want to drive in Brazil, you'll take more public transportation. You may be restricted to just one area of Brazil. We were very mobile. I don't recommend driving in Brazil. The roads are bad and the signage is almost non-present. Allow yourself some time to recover in between training sessions, and see Brazil! It's absolutely beautiful. The next trip we take will probable just be in two locations, a training city and a vacation city. Too much travel will bog you down and stress you out. Well, that's my Capoeira Over 40 Brazil trip.

I hope it has given you insight on scheduling and itinerary planning for your trip. Remember to read the whole travel blog at www.gingaandgrowstrong.com.

Axé!

Printed in Great Britain
by Amazon